9494
2017

Acknowledgments

The authors thank everyone who picked up one of the previous two editions of *Walking Los Angeles* and was inspired to get to know our dynamic, overwhelming, and often-beautiful city better. We feel lucky to have had the opportunity to update this guide after six years and add several of our new favorite neighborhoods to the mix. Erin is also grateful to Tony, West, and Avery for joining her on her expeditions.

—*Erin Mahoney Harris and Zach Behrens*

Authors' Note

The face of Los Angeles is constantly changing, particularly when it comes to residential and commercial architecture, so you may find on your journeys that certain businesses, landmarks, and features described in this book have changed since it was written. We encourage you to use our directions as a general guide but also to explore at a leisurely pace and make your own discoveries.

That said, we also implore you to use common sense to ensure your safety and comfort: bring a buddy if you're exploring a new neighborhood that you don't feel entirely at ease about visiting; walk during the day rather than at night; wear appropriate shoes to prevent blisters; keep dogs leashed at all times, as these are primarily urban routes close to street traffic; and, finally, if you're bringing a baby or child in a stroller, please pay attention to the difficulty rating to see if stairways are part of that route. (Note that routes with just a few steps here and there don't include the stairway notation.)

The boundaries mentioned at the beginning of each walk are meant to give you an idea of the major streets that surround the route to make it easier to find. These streets don't always appear on the accompanying maps, so you can look up the intersection indicated at the walk's starting point using GPS, a mapping app, a website, or a good old-fashioned paper map if you need help locating the beginning of your route. For walks that start within a mile of a Metro station, we've included that information as well.

Happy trekking!

Table of Contents

WALKING – – – – → LOS ANGELES

38 of the City's Most Vibrant Historic, Revitalized, and Up-and-Coming Neighborhoods

Third Edition

Erin Mahoney Harris with Zach Behrens

 WILDERNESS PRESS ... *on the trail since 1967*

Walking Los Angeles: 38 of the City's Most Vibrant Historic, Revitalized, and Up-and-Coming Neighborhoods

Copyright © 2017 by Erin Mahoney Harris and Zach Behrens
Project editor: Ritchey Halphen
Cartography: Scott McGrew and Tommy Hertzel; map data: OpenStreetMap
Cover design: Scott McGrew
Interior design: Lora Westberg
Cover and interior photos: Erin Mahoney Harris and Zach Behrens, unless otherwise noted
  (see page 217 for additional photo credits)
Copy editor: Kate Johnson
Proofreaders: Dan Downing, Rebecca Henderson
Indexer: Sylvia Coates

Library of Congress Cataloging-in-Publication Data

Names: Harris, Erin Mahoney, author. | Behrens, Zach, 1980– co-author.
Title: Walking Los Angeles : 38 of the city's most vibrant historic, revitalized, and up-and-coming
  neighborhoods / Erin Mahoney Harris and Zach Behrens.
Other titles: Walking LA | Walking Los Angeles
Description: 3rd edition. | Birmingham, AL : Wilderness Press, [2017]
Identifiers: LCCN 2016041687 | ISBN 978-0-89997-827-7 (paperback) | eISBN 978-0-89997-828-4
  (e-book)
Subjects: LCSH: Los Angeles (Calif.)—Guidebooks. | Walking—California—Los Angeles—Guidebooks.
  Historic sites—California—Los Angeles—Guidebooks. | Historic buildings—California—Los
  Angeles—Guidebooks. | Architecture—California—Los Angeles—Guidebooks. | Los Angeles
  (Calif.)—Buildings, structures, etc.—Guidebooks. | BISAC: TRAVEL / United States / West / Pacific
  (AK, CA, HI, NV, OR, WA). | SPORTS & RECREATION / Walking. | HEALTH & FITNESS / Healthy Living.
Classification: LCC F869.L83 H27 2017 | DDC 917.94/9404—dc23
LC record available at lccn.loc.gov/2016041687

Manufactured in the United States of America

Published by: **WILDERNESS PRESS**
              An imprint of AdventureKEEN
              2204 First Ave. S., Suite 102
              Birmingham, AL 35233
              800-443-7227, fax 205-326-1012

Visit wildernesspress.com for a complete list of our books and for ordering information. Contact us at our website, at facebook.com/wildernesspress1967, or at twitter.com/wilderness1967 with questions or comments. To find out more about who we are and what we're doing, visit blog.wildernesspress.com.

Distributed by Publishers Group West

Cover photo: Echo Park with the LA skyline in the distance (see Walk 26, page 123); Ian G Dagnall/Alamy Stock Photo

SAFETY NOTICE Although Wilderness Press and the authors have made every attempt to ensure that the information in this book is accurate at press time, they are not responsible for any loss, damage, injury, or inconvenience that may occur to anyone while using this book. You are responsible for your own safety and health while following the walking trips described here.

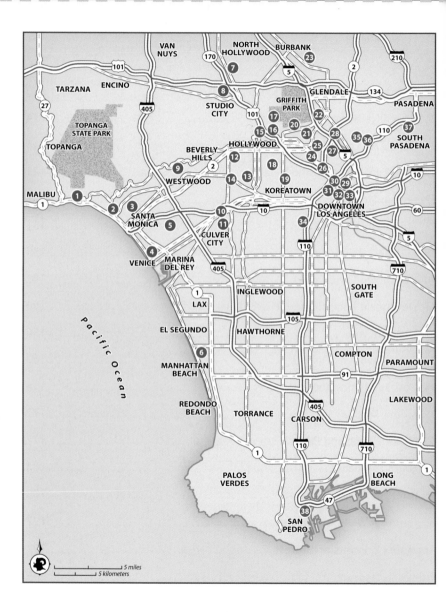

Introduction

Los Angeles has gotten a bad rap in the past. Sure, it's sprawling, traffic-choked, and smoggy. But the air continues to clear—you can see the mountains now!—and LA's public-transit options are growing like no other US city's. There's a public push and political will to make the city more walkable and bikeable. The backlog of crumpled sidewalks is being addressed, hundreds of miles of bike lanes are being added, and residents have taxed themselves to raise money for more trains.

So while LA has been a great place to walk for a while now, you can see it's only getting better. Really, it is—don't be deterred by our maze of freeways and pervasive car culture. No, you won't be able to traverse the greater metro area in a day, or even in a weekend, but take it in smaller doses and you'll be rewarded with a deeper understanding of this city's unique blend of culture, architecture, and topography.

Like the previous update, the third edition of this book continues to adapt to the changes Los Angeles is experiencing. We cut some walks and added others that we find to be especially charming or up-and-coming, such as Frogtown and the Downtown Arts District. This edition is also bound in a smaller format, so it's easier to carry around as you explore these rich neighborhoods. Finally, we hope the maps in this edition will be easier to use. Points of interest are now labeled on the map with the corresponding number found in the text and summary list.

The purpose of this book is to show that walking in LA can be an immensely rewarding experience, opening your eyes to hidden pockets that you never knew existed. These walks reflect the many faces of this fascinating city, and we hope that the discoveries you'll make as you explore the vibrant neighborhoods dotting its hills, valleys, and flatlands will encourage you to dust off your sneakers and leave the car in the garage at every opportunity.

Lake Shrine Temple, Self-Realization Fellowship (see facing page)

1 Castellammare in Pacific Palisades

BOUNDARIES: Pacific Coast Hwy., Sunset Blvd., Topanga State Park, Surfview Dr.
DISTANCE: About 1.25 miles
DIFFICULTY: Strenuous (includes stairways)
PARKING: Free street parking is available on Castellammare Dr.

This whimsically named neighborhood in the Pacific Palisades lies between the rolling green hills of Topanga State Park and the crashing surf of the Pacific Ocean—talk about exclusive real estate. Castellammare's lucky residents enjoy the soothing breezes and sweeping panoramas of the Pacific Ocean from their vantage point high in the hills. When money is no object, people tend to go nuts building their dream homes, making this an especially diverse neighborhood architecturally speaking. As you might expect on streets with names like Posetano and Tramonto, many of the homes are Mediterranean in style, but you'll also find a surprising hodgepodge of traditional, ranch-style, and modern houses in this rarefied coastal enclave.

Walk Description

Begin on Castellammare Drive, just southeast of Stretto Way, and walk north-west on Castellammare, past Stretto. At ❶ 17501, stop to admire the gorgeous Spanish-style home with colorful tile work. This stunner is the former abode of John Barrymore. Right next door is another Mediterranean-style home with elegantly carved wood trim; sunset views afforded by the row of windows on the second floor must be breathtaking.

Continue to where the paved road ends, and then go ahead on the dirt path. This pleasant, well-worn trail dips down toward PCH before heading back uphill to reconnect with the continuation of the paved street on what is still Castellammare Drive, passing a stairway on your right.

Climb the next stairway you come to on your right, near the intersection of Breve Way, enjoying the sounds of crashing surf behind you.

Turn right on Revello Drive at the top of the stairs. At the intersection of Posetano Road, you'll see a staircase heading about two-thirds of the way up the hill before it dead-ends in the brush. If you're looking for an extra workout, head up and down the steps a few times to get your heart pumping.

Nearby and Notable

The Self-Realization Fellowship's gorgeous flagship **Lake Shrine Temple,** at 17190 Sunset Blvd., about 0.3 mile north of Sunset's intersection with Castellammare Drive, is absolutely worth a visit. The lake and surrounding gardens provide numerous spots to sit and meditate or simply to enjoy the peaceful, lush surroundings. The ornate temple overlooking the grounds blends Eastern and Western architectural styles to stunning effect. The gardens, lake, and visitor center are open to the public Tuesday–Sunday; call 310-454-4114 for visiting hours. (To learn more about the Self-Realization Fellowship, see Mount Washington, page 172.)

Turn right on Posetano Road.

Look for a staircase on your right just before the road ends, and descend back to Castellammare Drive.

Turn left at the bottom of the stairs, and retrace your steps along Castellammare, crossing the dirt path once again. When the paved road begins, follow it all the way to Stretto Way.

Turn left on Stretto Way and follow the road as it winds up the hill.

Turn right on Posetano Road. At 17531 Posetano, you'll see a towering Italian-style villa named ❷ **Castillo del Mar.** The home's garage was the site of movie star Thelma Todd's mysterious death from carbon monoxide poisoning in 1935.

Ascend the staircase on your left just before 17445 Posetano. The long stairway is pleasantly bordered by bougainvillea, succulents, cacti, and wildflowers.

Turn right on Revello Drive at the top of the steps, and follow the road as it curves around to the left.

Bear left onto Tramonto Drive at the intersection. Watch out for cars because this street is a little more heavily traveled and there are no sidewalks. A gorgeous view of the ocean will open on your left as you continue up the road.

A Castellammare garden overlooks the ocean.

Turn right on Quadro Vecchio Drive. In contrast to the predominance of Mediterranean homes in the lower portion of the neighborhood, this street is populated by mostly ranch-style houses, with the exception of a striking modern structure at 266 Quadro Vecchio.

Turn left on Bellino Drive and continue to the intersection of Tramonto Drive.

Turn left on Tramonto and continue back to Revello Drive.

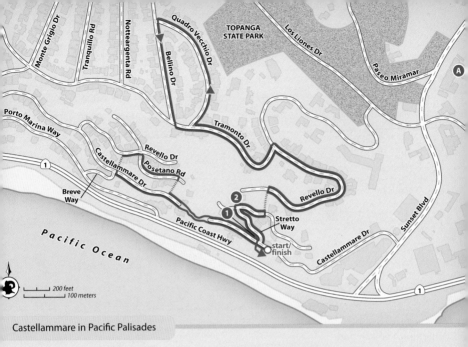

Castellammare in Pacific Palisades

Points of Interest

1. Former John Barrymore House 17501 Castellammare Drive, Los Angeles, CA 90272
2. Castillo del Mar (former Thelma Todd House) 17531 Posetano Road, Los Angeles, CA 90272

"Nearby and Notable," page 3:

A. Lake Shrine Temple, Self-Realization Fellowship 17190 Sunset Blvd., Los Angeles, CA 90272; 310-454-4114, yogananda-srf.org

Bear right to retrace your steps along Revello Drive. Continue all the way back to the last staircase you ascended, which you'll find on your left just past some towering bamboo.

Head down the stairs and turn right on Posetano Road, continuing to retrace your steps back to Stretto Way.

Bear left to go back down Stretto Way.

Turn left on Castellammare, heading back to your starting point.

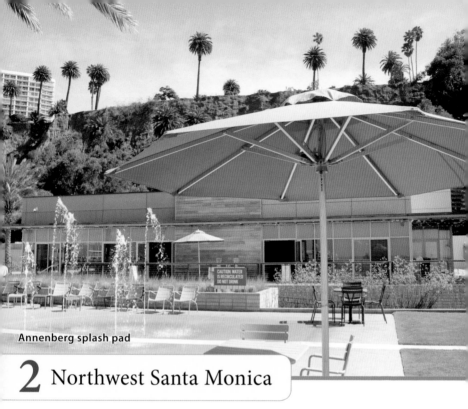

Annenberg splash pad

2 Northwest Santa Monica

BOUNDARIES: Pacific Ocean, Montana Ave., Seventh St., Entrada Dr.
DISTANCE: About 3 miles
DIFFICULTY: Strenuous (includes stairways)
PARKING: Free street parking is available on Fourth St., but please read posted signs for parking restrictions.

This walk offers a respectable workout in true Santa Monica style. Starting at the popular Santa Monica stairs on the northern border of the beach city, the route then drops down to the beach for a sun-drenched stroll to the popular Annenberg Community Beach House.

Note: While most of the walks in this book are designed to cover as much new ground as possible, this one returns to the starting point by more or less the same route. However, because most of that route overlooks the ocean or traverses the beach, we figured our readers wouldn't mind retracing their steps.

Walk Description

Begin at the intersection of Fourth Street and Adelaide Drive, right at the northernmost border of the city of Santa Monica in the exclusive residential neighborhood known as North of Montana.

Directly across the intersection, on the north side of Adelaide, is one of the two sets of Santa Monica stairs, a popular exercise destination for locals. Descend the long, narrow staircase all the way to Entrada Drive.

Turn right at the bottom of the stairs and follow the sidewalk, passing Canyon Charter School, a public elementary school in one of LA's most exclusive neighborhoods, on your left.

At the intersection with Amalfi Drive, look for the second set of stairs on your right, and ascend. The wooden staircase is wider than the first, making it easier to share with the remarkably fit locals trotting doggedly up and down.

Turn right at the top of the stairs, and follow Adelaide for a little under 0.5 mile down to Ocean Avenue, passing a succession of huge multimillion-dollar homes—the sprawling shingled Craftsman at 236 Adelaide is particularly envy-inducing.

When you reach Ocean Avenue, cross the street to ❶ **Palisades Park,** which is known informally as "The Bluffs" and stretches for more than 1.5 miles from Adelaide all the way down to Colorado Avenue. The long, narrow green space, shaded by eucalyptus, olive, pine, and palm trees, offers stunning views of Santa Monica Bay that encompass Palos Verdes Peninsula, Catalina Island, the Santa Monica Pier, and Point Dume in Malibu. Here, at the northernmost end of the park, you'll notice a charming totem pole, picnic tables, and a small grove of fragrant eucalyptus trees.

Turn left to walk through the park. You have your choice of dirt paths: the one closer to the street is shaded by pine trees, while the one on the ocean side is sunnier but offers spectacular views. On the green space between the two paths, you'll likely see trainers leading fitness classes. The practice is so popular, in fact, that the city of

Santa Monica cracked down in recent years, requiring trainers to obtain a permit to conduct sessions in city parks to keep them from being overrun with fitness enthusiasts. You'll pass through a pretty rose garden across from the intersection with Palisades Avenue and then come to an interesting spherical wooden sculpture just south of the garden.

Shortly thereafter, across from the intersection of Montana Avenue, you'll reach the staircase that will take you down to the beach on your right. Descend the long stairway, cross the bridge over the Pacific Coast Highway, and then continue down the spiral staircase to a beach parking lot.

Cross the lot toward the beach. On your left, you'll pass a private beach club and a public swing set.

Turn right when you reach the beach path. Around this point, the path goes from being exclusively for cyclists to being a shared pedestrian/bike path. It's wise to keep right to make way for passing cyclists.

Continue on the beach path a little under 0.5 mile to ❷ **Back on the Beach Cafe.** Just past the café is a boardwalk, which you can follow to the left if you'd like to spend some meditative moments on one of the thoughtfully provided benches looking out over the ocean.

Follow the boardwalk to the right toward the ❸ **Annenberg Community Beach House.** This facility opened in 2009 as an alternative to the private beach clubs and homes that monopolize nearly all of the oceanfront real estate in these parts. The beach house features a lovely pool and facilities that are open to the public during the summer for a modest day-use fee, as well as areas open to the public at no charge. These include a small children's play area next to Back on the Beach Cafe and, just north of the pool, a picnic area with tables, umbrellas, and a splash pad for kids to play around in. North of the beach house is the historic Marion Davies Guest House, now open for occasional public tours and used to host special events.

After checking out the facilities, retrace your steps back down the beach path, across the pedestrian bridge, and up the stairway to Palisades Park.

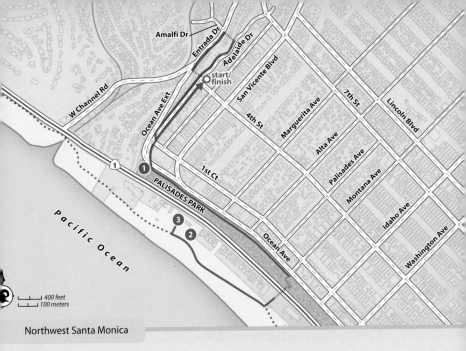

Northwest Santa Monica

Points of Interest

1. **Palisades Park** Ocean Avenue between Colorado Avenue and Adelaide Drive, Santa Monica, CA 90402

2. **Back on the Beach Cafe** 445 Pacific Coast Highway, Santa Monica, CA 90402; 310-393-8282, backonthebeachcafe.com

3. **Annenberg Community Beach House** 415 Pacific Coast Highway, Santa Monica, CA 90402; 310-458-4904, annenbergbeachhouse.com

Head back the way you came through the park.

Turn right onto Adelaide when you come to the end of the park, carefully crossing the street. Note that the road splits here as it turns to head east—make sure to take the upper road on your right to get onto Adelaide instead of following the lower Ocean Avenue Extension on the left.

Follow Adelaide back to your starting point at the intersection of Fourth Street.

Playing on a Moreton Bay fig tree

3 Northeast Santa Monica and Brentwood

BOUNDARIES: Montana Ave., 17th St., La Mesa Dr., 26th St.
DISTANCE: About 3 miles
DIFFICULTY: Easy
PARKING: Free street parking is available on 17th St., but please read posted signs for parking restrictions.

This route travels the northernmost reaches of the city of Santa Monica before briefly crossing into the LA neighborhood of Brentwood to check out the rustic-looking yet upscale Brentwood Country Mart shopping center. But the main draw of this area has nothing to do with retail, but rather what very well may be the most incredible trees you've ever seen. The quiet residential La Mesa Drive was planted with Moreton Bay fig trees back in the 1920s (rumor has it the saplings were mistaken for magnolias) that have since grown to mammoth yet regal proportions, offering a special horticultural treat that visitors to this wealthy enclave can marvel at from the sidewalk.

Walk Description

Begin on 17th Street just north of Montana Avenue. ❶ **Sweet Lady Jane,** renowned purveyor of all things sugary and delicious, anchors the northwest corner of the intersection. Start walking northwest away from Montana along the pretty, magnolia-lined street. The houses—predominantly Spanish in style with some traditional homes thrown in—range in size from modest to palatial and boast a mix of manicured lawns and tasteful, drought-tolerant landscaping.

Right after you cross Carlyle Avenue, a couple of houses on the right stand out: a large, boxy Spanish home with pretty tile work adorning the second story and a wood-paneled home with a stone chimney and sloped roof that brings to mind a ski lodge. Another interesting structure appears on the left as you approach the intersection with Georgina Avenue; this one is almost fortresslike, with its plain stucco walls and high windows, and it has a cool domed metal kids' climbing structure in the front yard.

Turn right on San Vicente Boulevard. Twisted coral trees line the median of the wide boulevard, blooming bright reddish orange in the spring.

Look for the crosswalk at the intersection with 19th Street, and cross over to the north side of San Vicente. Here the street becomes La Mesa Drive, home to those magnificent Moreton Bay fig trees. Follow La Mesa as it curves to the right.

With their massive trunks, snaking roots, and twisting limbs, the trees almost appear to be primordial. Their canopies spread out to keep the street permanently shaded, and in the summer, the sidewalks become littered with their fallen fruit. Perhaps the most fascinating feature of the Moreton Bay fig is its roots, which on some trees reach chest-high. It's almost impossible to resist hopping up and walking along them, balance beam–style, following their meandering path around the base of the tree, so have a little fun and go for it. While arboreal enthusiasts will likely be too caught up by the trees to notice, architecture buffs will appreciate the range in styles of the uniformly enormous homes on this street: Tudor, Spanish, modern, French château, Cape Cod, Tuscan villa—really quite a mix.

About halfway down the block, keep your eyes peeled in front of the home at 2209 La Mesa; you'll notice a whimsical etching of a castle and a mountain in the sidewalk.

Cross 24th Street and then keep right at the split in the road to follow La Mesa Way.

You'll pass under the thick branch of one last Moreton Bay fig before turning right on 26th Street.

Cross San Vicente Boulevard and then cross again to the east side of the street, turning right to continue south on 26th.

You will presently come to the ❷ **Brentwood Country Mart.** The distinctive red clapboard structure, built in 1948, houses a collection of upscale boutiques, a barber shop, a toy store, and both casual and upscale eateries, all arranged around a central courtyard with picnic tables and quarter-operated rides for the kids. Notable food purveyors here include the Farmshop market, restaurant, and bakery and Sweet Rose Creamery, which churns out delectable ice cream in both classic and unexpected flavors.

After you've explored the Country Mart, continue south on 26th Street until you come to Georgina Avenue, where you'll turn right and leave the busy commercial street behind to return to bucolic residential surroundings—bucolic, that is, apart from the seemingly ongoing construction that seems to occur in upscale neighborhoods like this one.

Turn left on 23rd Street, enjoying the pleasing variety of foliage and interesting amalgams of residential architecture. The home at 624 23rd St. is particularly notable, its curved roof reminiscent of the inverted hull of a boat.

Turn right on Alta Avenue, enjoying the alpine scent of the pine trees lining the sidewalk.

Turn left on 17th Street to return to your starting point just north of Montana Avenue.

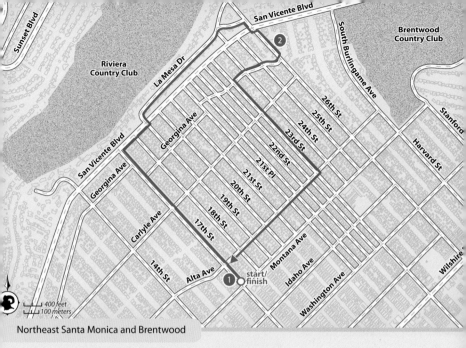

Northeast Santa Monica and Brentwood

Points of Interest

 Sweet Lady Jane 1631 Montana Ave., Santa Monica, CA 90403; 310-254-9499, sweetladyjane.com

2 **Brentwood Country Mart** 225 26th St., Santa Monica, CA 90402; 310-451-9877, brentwoodcountrymart.com

Venice canals

4 Venice Beach

BOUNDARIES: Abbot Kinney Blvd., Pacific Ave., Washington Blvd.
DISTANCE: About 2.25 miles
DIFFICULTY: Easy
PARKING: Free street parking is available on Ocean Avenue

Venice Beach may be the most distinctive beach town in all of Southern California thanks to its charming canals, which were built by real estate magnate Abbot Kinney in 1904 as an homage to the Venice in Italy. Unlike some other Westside neighborhoods, Venice Beach is more funky than fussy. That's not to say that the people who live here, particularly in the areas that line the canals and the oceanfront, aren't affluent, but it's more affordable than Santa Monica next door, and one might argue that it has a good deal more personality as well. All that said, the neighborhood is just as susceptible to gentrification as any other: home prices have soared in recent years, and high-priced retailers have moved into the shopping districts. Nonetheless, the boho vibe is still very much alive and well.

Note: This walk can be particularly fun for both you and your pooch, provided it doesn't get overexcited at the sight of ducks. If you do bring a dog, resist the temptation to remove its leash during the canal portion of the walk. Toward the end of the route, you'll come to the Westminster Off-Leash Dog Park, where Rover can get footloose and fancy-free with his canine pals.

Walk Description

This excursion begins in the South Venice neighborhood, at the intersection of Venice Boulevard and Ocean Avenue. Begin by walking south on Ocean Avenue toward Linnie Avenue. Notice that the homes along this stretch of Ocean are all relatively modest in size and style, although one can't help but wonder how long until these small dwellings are torn down and replaced with boxy mini-mansions, as seems to be happening in so many other Westside neighborhoods.

Turn right on Linnie Avenue.

Cross the bridge arching over the Eastern Canal, pausing on top to admire the interesting mix of homes lining the waterway. The houses here are decidedly grander than those on Ocean Avenue, ranging in architectural style from American Colonial Revival to modern to Tudor Revival.

On the other side of the bridge, make an immediate left to follow the sidewalk along the canal.

Follow the sidewalk as it turns right, taking you along Howland Canal. Ducks are everywhere, quackily going about their business, and small boats and canoes are docked in front of some houses. The homes along this waterway are all beautifully maintained, and each is distinct. Notable architectural styles here include Craftsman, Spanish Colonial Revival, Cape Cod, and modern stucco beach homes with huge picture windows.

Cross Dell Avenue and then pause in the shade of a giant pine tree adorned with hanging glass lanterns to bask in the tranquil, salt-tinged air of this remarkable neighborhood. It's an interesting mélange, this blend of old-world Italy and funky SoCal beach-culture lifestyle.

Follow the sidewalk as it turns right at the corner of Grand Canal.

Turn right to follow the sidewalk alongside Linnie Canal.

Shortly after turning the corner, cross the pedestrian bridge on your left to the other side of the waterway, and then turn right to continue walking next to Linnie Canal. After crossing Dell Avenue, on your left you'll see Linnie Canal Park, a small playground complete with a dedicated duck habitat. Residents manage to do quite a lot with their relatively small amount of lot space. You'll see edible gardens, majestic shade trees, and notable sculptures adorning front yards along this stretch.

At the end of Linnie Canal, turn left to follow the sidewalk and you'll notice two unusually large residences on your left, one on each side of the alley. These matching structures look like something out of an Austrian village and appear to be the largest homes on the canals.

Turn left to follow the sidewalk alongside Carroll Canal.

Turn right on Dell Avenue. When you reach South Venice Boulevard, you'll spot a colorful mural depicting canal community life on the southwest corner.

Turn right on South Venice Boulevard and follow the sycamore-shaded sidewalk for a little under 0.5 mile to Abbot Kinney Boulevard. The ❶ **Venice Farmers Market** sets up in the parking lot in the median of South Venice Boulevard between Dell Avenue and Ocean Avenue on Fridays, 7–11 a.m.

Turn left on Abbot Kinney. This street has become a foodie's dream in recent years with an influx of farm-to-table establishments like ❷ **The Tasting Kitchen** and ❸ **Gjelina.** If, however, you're hungry for a tasty but decidedly more casual bite, you can't go wrong with ❹ **Lemonade,** back on the corner of Abbot Kinney and Venice Boulevards.

Back Story: Venice of America Amusement Park

The area now known as Venice was originally founded as Venice of America by Abbot Kinney in the fledgling years of the 20th century. This themed resort town was built on reclaimed marshland and featured an amusement park, a heated indoor saltwater "plunge," a miniature railroad, and more than 16 miles of canals, complete with Venetian gondolas and gondoliers. Unfortunately, expensive upkeep and the rise of the automobile meant that most of the canals were paved over by 1929, and the remaining six eventually fell into disrepair. Fortunately, those six were restored in the early 1990s, and today the neighborhood built around the canals is affluent and idyllic.

Continue along Abbot Kinney for 0.75 mile. This trendy shopping district pretty much exemplifies gentrification. While Abbot Kinney used to be decidedly quirky—some might even have called it gritty—the street's bungalow storefronts now specialize in upscale casual-chic clothing, furnishings, and decor. In other words, if you're looking for a crocheted bikini or a $100 hoodie, you've come to the right place.

Just before you reach Westminster Avenue, notice the low brick structure on the left with a faded metal sign that reads IRV'S FAMILY MARKET. The distinguished old building now houses art galleries and shops.

On the final block of Abbot Kinney, between Westminster Avenue and Main Street, you'll come across ❺ The Cook's Garden by HGEL, a nursery and garden-supply shop that supplies produce to area restaurants. Westminster Avenue Elementary School is across the street on your left.

Turn left on Main Street. This leg of the walk is a little drab compared with the thriving consumer mecca you left behind on Abbot Kinney but is punctuated with colorful murals. As you approach the corner of Westminster Avenue, you'll see the

6 **Westminster Off-Leash Dog Park** on your right. This is a good place to stop if you've brought your pooch along.

Cross Westminster and continue on Main Street about two blocks to the Windward Circle roundabout, which was a picturesque lagoon back in Kinney's day, when more than 16 miles of canals snaked through the Venice of America.

At this point, you may choose to turn right on Windward Avenue, which will take you the few short blocks to the Venice Beach Boardwalk. Also known as Ocean Front Walk, this is a popular destination for tourists, skaters, and cyclists who like to cruise the waterfront. Sidewalk vendors hawk incense, T-shirts, and various tourist-targeted wares of questionable value. If you do take this detour, return the way you came to the corner of Main Street and Windward.

Walk south along the west side of the rotary to remain on Main Street.

Turn left on Venice Way and walk about a third of a mile.

Venice Way curves and becomes Ocean Avenue. Continue on Ocean Avenue to reach your starting point near the intersection of Linnie Avenue.

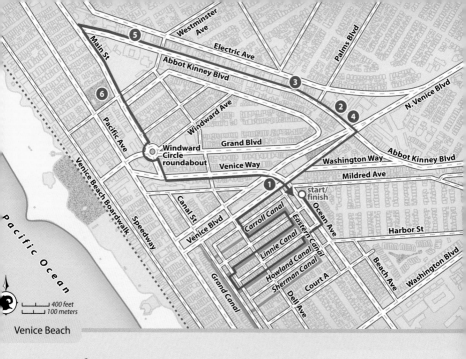

Venice Beach

400 feet
100 meters

Points of Interest

1 **Venice Farmers Market** Corner of Dell Avenue and South Venice Boulevard, Los Angeles, CA 90291; Fridays, 7–11 a.m.

2 **The Tasting Kitchen** 1633 Abbot Kinney Blvd., Los Angeles, CA 90291; 310-392-6644, thetastingkitchen.com

3 **Gjelina** 1429 Abbot Kinney Blvd., Los Angeles, CA 90291; 310-450-1429, gjelina.com

4 **Lemonade** 1661 Abbot Kinney Blvd., Los Angeles, CA 90291; 310-452-6200, lemonadela.com/locations/westside/venice

5 **The Cook's Garden by HGEL** 1033 Abbot Kinney Blvd., Los Angeles, CA 90291; 310-944-1151, groedibles.com

6 **Westminster Off-Leash Dog Park** 1234 Pacific Ave., Los Angeles, CA 90291; 310-310-1550, venicedogpark.org

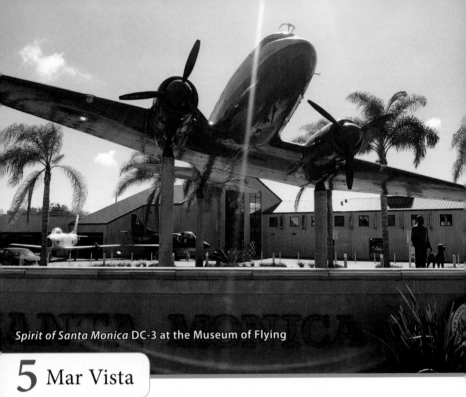

Spirit of Santa Monica DC-3 at the Museum of Flying

5 Mar Vista

BOUNDARIES: National Blvd., Bundy Dr./Centinela Ave., Palms Blvd., McLaughlin Ave./
Barrington Ave. (*Note:* Certain streets change names along the route.)
DISTANCE: About 2.5 miles
DIFFICULTY: Moderate (includes stairway and hills)
PARKING: Free parking is available at Airport Park.

This walk begins in the southeast corner of Santa Monica at Airport Park before crossing the border into the neighborhood of Mar Vista to travel up and down the stairs and hills of this pleasant enclave, which is fast becoming another Westside hot spot for both prospective home buyers and interesting new retailers and restaurants.

Walk Description

Begin at ❶ **Airport Park,** on the grounds of the Santa Monica Airport. The park, located adjacent to the tarmac, includes a soccer field; a sandy playground; an open, grassy field; and an off-leash dog area. The ❷ **Museum of Flying** and the casual ❸ **Spitfire Grill** are located nearby. It's a fun place to hang out, especially if you're interested in watching prop planes (and the occasional private jet) taxiing down the runway for takeoff to the west and coming in for landing from the east.

Follow the sidewalk east toward Bundy Drive. If you're a fan of canines, you can follow the path past the dog area that leads to a ramp up to the street; otherwise, just take the sidewalk adjacent to Airport Avenue.

Turn right to head south on Bundy. This stretch of sidewalk is sunny and located alongside a busy street, but you only need to walk here for 0.2 mile.

Cross to the east side of the street at Rose Avenue, and follow the driveway uphill toward the site of Ocean View Farms, a community garden with a multiyear waiting list. You'll cut across the parking lot to head toward the baseball fields, passing the snack bar and bleachers to find a dirt path cutting across a field toward a gate in the fence on the other side of the property. The gate should be unlocked and open during daylight hours.

After passing through the gate, you'll find yourself on Grand View Boulevard. The intersection with Indianapolis Street is just to your left. Head straight down Indianapolis. When you reach the intersection of Keeshen Drive, you'll notice two large, newly constructed modern homes on either side of the street. They stand in stark contrast to many of the older, more modest-sized homes in the neighborhood and illustrate the rapid gentrification of this prized neighborhood adjacent to Santa Monica.

When you reach Inglewood Boulevard, you'll get a great view of the Getty Center and the Westwood Corridor skyline to the north. Cross Inglewood and turn right.

After passing two houses, you'll come to the Mar Vista Stairs, a public stairway leading down to the street below (just past 3296 Inglewood Blvd.). Descend the stairs and your vista expands to include Griffith Observatory, the HOLLYWOOD sign, and downtown Los Angeles with the San Gabriel Mountains beyond. To the right you'll see Baldwin Hills.

Turn right on Granville Avenue at the bottom of the stairs. You'll pass Mar Vista Elementary School on your left. The school is decorated with cute, colorful murals and tile work.

Turn left on Woodbine Street. Look left as you cross Stoner Avenue, and you'll notice a rusty old Cold War (or possibly World War II)–era air-raid siren about half-way down the block.

Turn right on Federal Avenue and walk one block.

Turn left on Palms Boulevard and walk one more block.

Cross McLaughlin Avenue and turn left. The grounds of the ❹ **Mar Vista Recreation Center** are on your right, and you'll pass a series of kinetic-exercise machines located alongside a dirt path, free and available to the frugal and fitness-minded public.

Continue northwest on McLaughlin. The liquidambar trees lining this curving stretch of road make it one of the relatively few thoroughfares in Los Angeles where you can experience fall color.

At the intersection with Indianapolis Street/Federal Avenue, cross the street to turn left on Indianapolis.

Cross Granville Avenue when Indianapolis dead-ends, and you'll see the Mar Vista Stairs you descended earlier just to your left. Ascend the staircase.

At the top, turn right on Inglewood and follow the road as it heads downhill, enjoying the view that opens up to include Century City to the east and the Santa Monica Mountains to the west. The flight path of Santa Monica Airport is directly ahead, so you may see some planes coming in for landing.

Walk a few short blocks to Stanwood Drive and turn left. Now it's time to head back uphill, but you'll be rewarded at the crest with a view of the ocean.

Continue back down the hill until you reach Bundy Drive, and turn right.

Walk one block on Bundy to Airport Avenue and then turn left to cross at the intersection.

Follow Airport Avenue back to where you started at Airport Park.

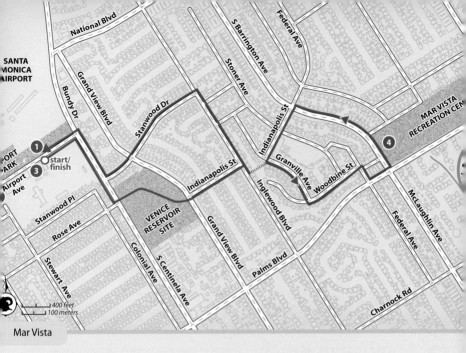

Mar Vista

Points of Interest

1 **Airport Park** 3201 Airport Ave., Santa Monica, CA 90405

2 **Museum of Flying** 3100 Airport Ave., Santa Monica, CA 90405; 310-398-2500, museumofflying.org

3 **Spitfire Grill** 3300 Airport Ave., Santa Monica, CA 90405; 310-397-3455, spitfiregrill.net

4 **Mar Vista Recreation Center** 11430 Woodbine St., Los Angeles, CA 90066; 310-398-5982, laparks.org/reccenter/mar-vista

Conqueror of the sand dune!

6 Manhattan Beach

BOUNDARIES: Rosecrans Ave., Blanche Rd., Manhattan Beach Blvd., Pacific Ocean
DISTANCE: About 2.5 miles
DIFFICULTY: Easy
PARKING: Free street parking is available on Bell Avenue.

One of the South Bay's wealthiest cities, Manhattan Beach in many ways presents more of an Orange County vibe than an LA one. Popular with families for its strong school district and with everyone for its stunning seaside location and all-around pleasantness, this beach town is more laid-back than Santa Monica but decidedly more upscale than Venice.

Walk Description

Begin at ❶ **Sand Dune Park.** This neighborhood gem features a small playground in addition to the eponymous 100-foot sand hill that many locals climb for an effective if punishing workout. If you're not in the mood for trudging up a giant wall of sand—which, because of its popularity, requires an online reservation to climb for adults (kids are welcome to climb without one)—the park's shaded stairways and sidewalks offer a pleasant meandering path on which to explore your surroundings.

Walk southeast on Bell Avenue, away from the park, passing a schoolyard on the right.

Turn right on 24th Street and head uphill. This residential area, known as the Gas Lamp Section, features adorable houses squeezed together on fairly small lots, much like many SoCal seaside communities. You'll pass the front of Grand View Elementary School before reaching the top of the hill, which affords an expansive view of the ocean a few blocks ahead.

Turn right on Highland Avenue and walk one block to 25th Street.

Cross Highland at the sidewalk and then follow the 25th Street walkway all the way down to the Strand, as the beachside pedestrian/bicycle path is called throughout the South Bay beach cities. At this point, the pedestrian walkway is completely separate from the Marvin Braude Bike Trail, which is a few steps down below next to the sand, making for a pleasant stroll unimpeded by two-wheelers.

Turn left to follow the Strand a little under 0.75 mile to the ❷ **Manhattan Beach Pier,** which you'll see prettily framed up ahead with the Palos Verdes Peninsula as a backdrop. You'll pass impressive beachfront homes on your left, and the median on your right features lovely water-wise landscaping, with ice plant, California poppies, and agave. You'll see plenty of volleyball nets set up down on the sand—the city hosts the popular Manhattan Beach Open volleyball tournament every summer.

When you reach the pier, you may choose to walk its length of about 900 feet to reach the distinctive Roundhouse at the far end, which houses a small aquarium, typically open in the afternoons on weekdays and all day on weekends. Admission to the Roundhouse Aquarium is free, although donations are welcomed.

After visiting the pier, head east on Manhattan Beach Boulevard, climbing uphill past the touristy shops and restaurants.

Turn left on Highland Avenue, passing pricey boutiques as well as enduringly popular restaurants such as ❸ The Kettle, ❹ The Izaka-ya by Katsu-ya, and ❺ Uncle Bill's Pancake House.

Turn right when you reach Uncle Bill's onto 13th Street. You'll pass the police department on your left and Shade, a boutique hotel, on your right. You may choose to explore the plaza around Shade, which features a mosaic fountain, a neat wind sculpture, and, if you venture in a little farther, several more restaurants.

Turn left on Valley Drive.

Cross 15th Street and then cross Valley Drive to reach the grassy meridian. This wide center island features a tree-shaded walkway known as Veterans Parkway.

Turn left to follow the wood-chip walking path down the center of the meridian, passing the sports fields and playgrounds of Live Oak Park on your left. Keep an eye out for a sculpture titled *A Wave for the Future,* which houses a time capsule placed by the Manhattan Beach Leadership Class of 2000. The scent of the eucalyptus and conifers planted along the parkway gives it a pleasant woodsy feel even though you're less than 0.25 mile from the beach.

When you reach Blanche Road, follow the stairway on your left down to the street, and then cross the street to head north on Blanche.

Cross 25th Street and continue straight ahead on Bell Avenue. Follow Bell back to your starting point near Sand Dune Park.

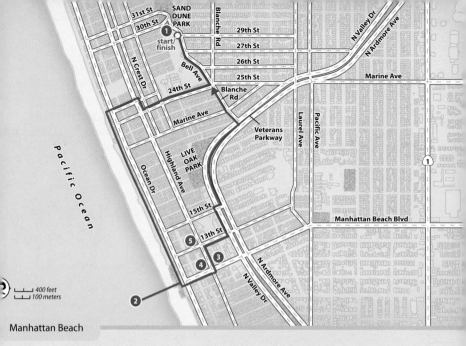

Points of Interest

1. **Sand Dune Park** Bell Avenue, Manhattan Beach, CA 90266; 310-802-5410

2. **Manhattan Beach Pier/Roundhouse Aquarium** Western end of Manhattan Beach Blvd., Manhattan Beach, CA 90266; 310-379-8117

3. **The Kettle** 1138 Highland Ave., Manhattan Beach, CA 90266; 310-545-8511, thekettle.net

4. **The Izaka-ya by Katsu-ya** 1133 Highland Ave., Manhattan Beach, CA 90266; 310-796-1888, katsu-yagroup.com/manhattan-beach

5. **Uncle Bill's Pancake House** 1305 Highland Ave., Manhattan Beach, CA 90266; 310-545-5177, unclebills.net

Entrance to the Academy of Television Arts and Sciences

7 NoHo Arts District

BOUNDARIES: Chandler Blvd., Vineland Ave., Tujunga Ave., Otsego St.
DISTANCE: About 0.5 mile
DIFFICULTY: Easy
PARKING: Metered parking is available on Lankershim Blvd.
NEAREST METRO STATION: Lankershim Blvd. and Chandler Blvd. (Red Line)

North Hollywood's Lankershim Boulevard was once hardly seen as a walking destination, but the birth of the NoHo Arts District makes it a neighborhood worth exploring. It's also a neighborhood still very much expanding: a stroll up and down the boulevard reveals it as a theatergoer's paradise, with 25 or so companies making their home here. And with numerous places catering to your food and drink needs, in addition to an eclectic array of public art splashed about, this is a great spot for a night out on the town.

Walk Description

Begin at the northeast corner of Lankershim Boulevard and Weddington Street. To the north you'll see NoHo Commons, a housing development and shopping center that was built in 2007 to take advantage of the Metro Red Line station at Chandler Boulevard. Head south on Lankershim.

At 5230 Lankershim you'll come upon a historic depot diner from the 1920s. It's currently home to ❶ **Sweetie Pie's NoHo,** part of the popular soul-food chain hailing from St. Louis and popularized by Oprah Winfrey. If you haven't already been tempted to stop for some ribs, hang a left at the driveway at 5220, home of the ❷ **Academy of Television Arts and Sciences** complex. Enter the main plaza, passing the colorful whirligigs that adorn the lawn next to the driveway entrance. The plaza is surrounded by bronze busts of famous personalities such as Red Skelton and Walt Disney, along with the unfamiliar faces of numerous company executives. The centerpiece is a massive burnished statue of the Emmy award, which sits atop a circular tiered fountain.

Exit the plaza via Blakeslee Avenue, which heads south to Magnolia Boulevard. Carefully cross Magnolia, a fairly busy street. The south side of Magnolia is home to several small theaters. The ❸ **NoHo Arts Center,** at 11136, is devoted to multicultural performance art and theater. This block is also heavy on dining choices, including two places that have become instant classics: ❹ **Republic of Pie,** serving artisanal pies, coffee, and tea, and ❺ **Eat,** a diner where breakfast rules and zucchini shreds are a popular accompaniment to omelets and such.

Continue west to Lankershim and make your way catty-corner, where ❻ **Pitfire Pizza Company** occupies an industrial-looking concrete building with an airy interior of exposed brick and corrugated metal. A sign proclaims the pizza joint's mission of "Feeding a Hungry Nation." This is an excellent place to stop for a bite of mouthwatering wood-fired pizzas with innovative toppings, or a delectable soup or sandwich. You can dine inside to enjoy the aroma of fresh-baked pizza crust or outside to relax on the pleasant patio. Next door to Pitfire is another public art display: a colorful mural depicting an idyllic park scene by artist Tim Fields.

Just north of Pitfire, the collection of shops, galleries, and restaurants features colorful neon and metal signs that compete for the attention of passersby, as well as a former alleyway–turned–pedestrian plaza. This is one of LA's so-called People Streets, a reclaiming of public roads to make neighborhoods more pedestrian-friendly. This is a good spot to grab a chair and table and enjoy some coffee and read a book (say, study up for your next *Walking LA* adventure).

The delightfully garish entrance to ❼ **Tokyo Delve's Sushi Bar,** at 5239, features squiggly neon letters and metal cutouts of classic Cadillacs. The kooky exterior design is an indicator of the crazy experience that awaits within, where diners are encouraged to dance on their chairs as everyone joins in on '80s sing-alongs. This might be the only sushi bar in LA where a club-style line builds outside to get in.

❽ **El Portal Theatre** is located at 5269 Lankershim. Originally built in 1926 as a vaudeville theater, the venue features a beautiful neon sign and gilded box office, and it is now home to three live performance theaters. ❾ **The Federal Bar,** a restaurant and bar housed in a 1920s brick bank building, sits on the northwest corner of Lankershim and Weddington.

Cross Lankershim at Weddington to return to your starting point on the east side of the street.

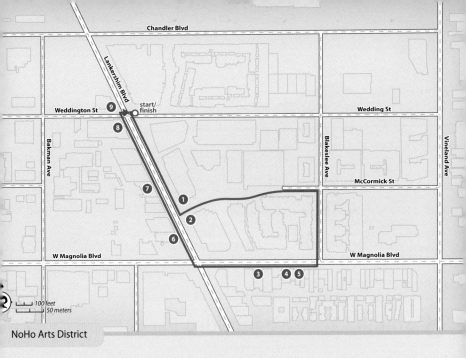

Points of Interest

1 **Sweetie Pie's NoHo** 5230 Lankershim Blvd., North Hollywood, CA 91601; 818-761-1325, sweetiepiesnoho.com

2 **Academy of Television Arts and Sciences** 5220 Lankershim Blvd., North Hollywood, CA 91601; 818-754-2800, emmys.com/academy

3 **NoHo Arts Center** 11136 Magnolia Blvd., North Hollywood, CA 91601; 818-508-7101, thenohoartscenter.com

4 **Republic of Pie** 11118 Magnolia Blvd., North Hollywood, CA 91601; 818-308-7990, republicofpie.com

5 **Eat** 11108 Magnolia Blvd., North Hollywood, CA 91601; 818-760-4787, eatnoho.com

6 **Pitfire Pizza Company** 5108 Lankershim Blvd., North Hollywood, CA 91601; 818-980-2949, pitfirepizza.com

7 **Tokyo Delve's Sushi Bar** 5239 Lankershim Blvd., North Hollywood, CA 91601; 818-766-3868, tokyodelvessushirestaurant.com

8 **El Portal Theatre** 5269 Lankershim Blvd., North Hollywood, CA 91601; 213-480-3232, elportaltheatre.com

9 **The Federal Bar** 5303 Lankershim Blvd., North Hollywood, CA 91601; 818-980-2555, thefederalbar.com

A groovy TV landmark

8 Studio City's Woodbridge Park

BOUNDARIES: Moorpark St., Tujunga Ave., Ventura Blvd., Vineland Ave.
DISTANCE: About 1.75 miles
DIFFICULTY: Easy
PARKING: Metered street parking is available on Tujunga Ave.

Woodbridge Park is a preternaturally idyllic residential neighborhood in Studio City. The streets are shaded with mature trees and lined with meticulously maintained traditional homes. Bordered by the Los Angeles River on the south, US 101 on the northeast, and Tujunga Avenue on the west, this charismatic slice of affluent small-town America is effectively isolated from the anonymous sprawl of the surrounding Valley. Further, a neighborhood park and the collection of shops, salons, and restaurants in Tujunga Village ensure that residents have little reason to leave their bucolic surroundings. It's no wonder the Brady Bunch chose to settle down here.

Walk Description

Begin at the corner of Tujunga Avenue and Moorpark Street, and head south toward Woodbridge Street. You're in the midst of Tujunga Village, a collection of neighborhood restaurants, shops, and salons that retains a distinctly small-town vibe. ❶ **Aroma Coffee & Tea Company,** at 4360 Tujunga, is a big draw on this stretch; its ample patio seating makes it a great spot for dog owners, and the sandwiches, pastries, and coffee served by the friendly staff are usually quite tasty. But for really good food, ❷ **Caioti Pizza Café** might be the better bet. Chef-owner Ed LaDou is famed for popularizing California-style pizza (thin-crust pies with innovative toppings), but the restaurant is best known for its mysteriously named "The" Salad, a concoction of romaine, watercress, Gorgonzola cheese, balsamic vinaigrette, and walnuts said to induce labor in moms-to-be. ❸ **Vitello's Italian Restaurant,** at 4349 Tujunga, is the infamous spot where actor Robert Blake dined with his wife, Bonny Lee Bakley, just before she was found murdered in Blake's car, which was parked on a nearby side street. On a lighter note, Tujunga Village also features boutiques and salons; taco stands; a gourmet food store; and ❹ **Two Roads Theater,** which presents plays, movies, and musical performances.

After you cross Woodbridge, Tujunga Avenue becomes a residential street lined with a mix of old and new apartment buildings. Tujunga is a main thoroughfare between Moorpark Street and Ventura Boulevard, so traffic can be steady during rush hour.

Turn left on Aqua Vista Street, leaving the traffic of Tujunga behind as you enter an orderly suburban paradise of quiet, smoothly paved streets, carefully mani-cured lawns, and charming cottage-style homes. The dominant architectural styles are traditional ranch homes and wooden farmhouses, but Woodbridge Park also features a number of English cottages and Spanish-style homes.

Turn right on Elmer Avenue. You'll notice a colorful Southwest-style house on the southeast corner of Elmer and Aqua Vista. This vibrant home, sheltered by pine trees and innovatively adorned with abstract metal sculptures, stands out from the more traditional homes on this block. Continue south on Elmer Avenue. Straight ahead, you can see the low, green hills of Studio City.

Turn left on Dilling Street. At 11222 Dilling is a familiar house: despite a new paint job and the addition of a low wall around the front yard, it will be instantly recog-nizable by members of a certain generation as the ❺ **Brady Bunch abode.** (Please respect the owner's privacy.) Dilling is cut off from surrounding streets to the south and the east by the channelized Los Angeles River, which residents and city officials hope to see revitalized someday as a 52-mile-long park.

Turn left to head north on Klump Avenue, just opposite the Brady house. The street is trimmed with eucalyptus, sycamore, and magnolia trees, whose ample shade provides welcome relief during hot Valley summers. A quaint stone cottage catches the eye at 4146 Klump. After crossing Aqua Vista, look for the owl statue perched atop the low, peaked roof of the garage at 4208 Klump.

Turn right on Acama Street and continue one block to Fair Avenue. On the northeast corner of Fair and Acama is a home with a beautiful, abstract stained-glass window facing Acama.

Turn left on Fair Avenue. A very 1960s-style apartment building resides at 4252 Fair, its colorful facade a jarring combination of stucco, wood, and stone.

Turn right on Valley Spring Lane. At this point, the neighborhood starts to have a more rustic feel, as the sidewalks disappear and split-rail fencing defines yards. The rural vibe is somewhat spoiled by the hum of the adjacent US 101, however, as you continue east.

Follow the road as it curves left, becoming Valley Spring Place. When you reach the dead end, you'll see a modern black, wood fence on the left, constructed to prevent cars from trying to cut through the narrow passageway leading to Fair Avenue. Cut through here, and continue south on Fair Avenue.

Turn right on Valley Spring Lane and continue one short block to Klump Avenue.

Turn right on Klump. At the end of the street, continue straight along the footpath that passes through a picket fence entryway.

The path emerges into the park for which this neighborhood is named. ❻ **Woodbridge Park** is a good-sized community-gathering place complete with a playground, recreation center, and jogging trails. Cut through the park, bearing left toward the southwest corner, where you will come upon the intersection of Elmer Avenue and Woodbridge Street.

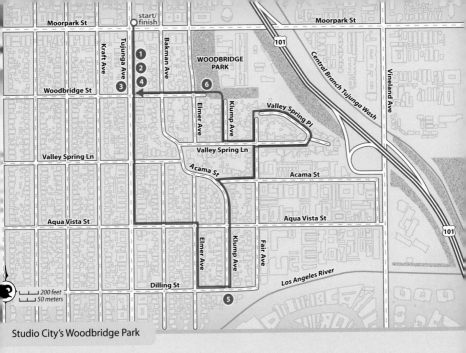

Studio City's Woodbridge Park

Points of Interest

1 Aroma Coffee & Tea Company 4360 Tujunga Ave., Studio City, CA 91604; 818-508-0677, aromacoffeeandtea.com

2 Caioti Pizza Café 4346 Tujunga Ave., Studio City, CA 91604; 818-761-3588, caiotipizzacafe.com

3 Vitello's Italian Restaurant 4349 Tujunga Ave., Studio City, CA 91604; 818-769-0905, vitellosrestaurant.com

4 Two Roads Theater 4348 Tujunga Ave., Studio City, CA 91604; 818-415-9568, tworoadstheater.com

5 Brady Bunch House 11222 Dilling St., Studio City, CA 91604

6 Woodbridge Park 11240 Moorpark St., Studio City, CA 91602; 818-769-4415, laparks.org/park/woodbridge

Head west on Woodbridge, back toward Tujunga Avenue. At the intersection of Bakman Avenue, you'll see an English cottage that looks like it belongs in the pages of a children's storybook.

Turn right on Tujunga Avenue, returning to your starting point in Tujunga Village.

Iconic Royce Hall is UCLA's performing-arts venue.

9 UCLA Campus in Westwood

BOUNDARIES: Sunset Blvd., Hilgard Ave., Le Conte Ave., Gayley Ave.
DISTANCE: About 1.75 miles
DIFFICULTY: Moderate (includes stairways)
PARKING: Limited street parking is available on Hilgard Ave. south of Sunset Blvd.
  Paid parking is available on campus.

UCLA is one of the best-known campuses in the famed University of California system. Renowned for its challenging academic programs as well as its gorgeous, ideally situated campus, UCLA represents the mythical undergraduate experience that many of us wish we'd had.

This route explores the most scenic spots on the large campus, taking in innovative artwork, classically beautiful architecture, and a lovely botanical garden that has evolved over several decades.

Walk Description

Begin on Hilgard Avenue, south of Sunset Boulevard and near the intersection with Charles E. Young Drive, which splits off from the west side of Hilgard. Follow Young Drive south into the UCLA campus.

Turn right at the semicircular driveway to head into the ❶ **Franklin D. Murphy Sculpture Garden.** This is the largest outdoor sculpture garden on the West Coast and one of the prettiest, with its rolling green lawns and feathery jacaranda trees. Pass a shallow fountain on the right as you descend the short stairway into the sunken grassy area. Notice the two columns topped with bronze sculptures of nude dancers by Robert Graham. The sculpture garden spans more than 5 acres of UCLA's north campus and includes an eclectic blend of naturalistic and sleekly modern pieces from artists such as Alexander Calder, Henri Matisse, Jacques Lipchitz, and Auguste Rodin. After taking some time to admire the sculptures and bas-reliefs, return to the eastern end of the garden and follow the sidewalk south.

As you head south along the sidewalk, on your right you'll come to ❷ **Bunche Hall,** which features an innovative indoor palm garden in its central atrium. Take a quick detour through the corridor past the atrium and out to the west side of the 12-story building to take in Maynard Lyndon's modern architecture. Built in 1964, Bunche Hall has been nicknamed "The Waffle" for its striking grid of three-dimensional square windows. Exit the way you came in, and then continue south along the sidewalk, passing Lu Valle Commons on your left.

When you reach Dodd Hall, turn right to follow the diagonal path through the sunken lawn of Dickson Court, which is shaded by mature sycamore and Moreton Bay fig trees.

After crossing Portola Plaza, the street that borders Dickson Court, you'll find yourself in the university's historic quad. This wide-open grassy area runs between the four original buildings of the Westwood campus, all of which were built in 1929 in the Italian Romanesque style. You'll pass Haines Hall on your right and Kinsey Hall on your left before coming to the campus's two best-known landmarks. On your right is the iconic ❸ **Royce Hall.** Designed by architect David Allison and based on a basilica in Milan, it houses UCLA's Center for the Art of Performance. Powell Library is on your left, and while it bears some architectural resemblance to Royce Hall, it was designed by another architect, George Kelham. Powell's octagonal tower and main entrance are modeled after two different churches in Italy. Part of what makes the northeast portion of the UCLA campus so beautiful is its architectural integrity; the redbrick Mediterranean-style buildings lend a distinguished, old-world feel to the College of Humanities.

Continue west through the quad, and you'll come to the semicircular Shapiro Fountain on Janss Terrace. Descend the Janss Steps, which served as the original entrance to the university, leading up from the former Westwood Boulevard. Admire the expansive view of the intramural fields stretched out in the distance. To your right is the ❹ **Fowler Museum at UCLA.** The Student Activities Center lies on the south side of the lawn below, with Kaufman Hall sitting opposite. On this side of campus, the university's newer buildings, with their redbrick and tan-stone exteriors, integrate beautifully with the original architecture.

Turn left at the bottom of the stairs, and follow the pathway heading south. Kerckhoff Hall lies straight ahead. Tree-shaded lawns roll gently alongside the sidewalk, providing yet another idyllic place for scholars to engage in or rest from their academic pursuits.

At the end of the sidewalk, turn right to follow the Bruin Walk into Bruin Plaza, home of the Bruin Bear, a 2-ton bronze statue of a ferocious-looking grizzly. At the southeast corner of the plaza is the ❺ **Ackerman Union,** distinguished by the arched wooden beams atop the roof. The UCLA Store occupies the first floor of the building and offers just about anything a student would need to purchase, from groceries to clothing to plush toys to books. The union also offers various casual-dining options.

Head back the way you came on Bruin Walk, past Ackerman Union, and return toward Kerckhoff Hall. Built in 1931, this is the only building on campus in the Collegiate Gothic architectural style. Continue straight ahead up the steps, and then turn right. Cross through the outdoor dining patio between Kerckhoff Hall and Moore Hall, which is on your left.

Turn left on Portola Plaza; the Mathematical Sciences Building is on your right. You are now entering the more technical side of campus, which is not nearly as picturesque as the humanities section in terms of architecture.

Continue straight on Portola Plaza, passing Kinsey Pavilion on your left. This building houses several lecture halls and is notable for the pretty mosaics in muted colors that adorn the top of its facade. Past Kinsey, you'll come to an open plaza with a beautiful inverted fountain in the center. A fairly new complex, the Evelyn and Mo Ostin Music Center, is located on the east side of the fountain.

Continue past the Ostin Music Center and then cut down the path on your right, which passes between a toddler play area and Franz Hall and takes you down to Charles E. Young Drive.

Turn right on Young Drive. As you approach the intersection with Manning Drive, you'll pass a pleasant, drought-tolerant rock garden on your right and see the large redbrick-and-glass Terasaki Life Sciences Building up ahead on your left.

Just before reaching Tiverton Drive, you'll see a ramp leading into the **6 Mildred E. Mathias Botanical Garden,** on your left. Follow the ramp down into the gardens. *Note:* At the time of writing, this was a newly built entrance to the gardens, which were still undergoing major improvements thanks to a $5 million gift from UCLA alumnus and philanthropist Morton La Kretz.

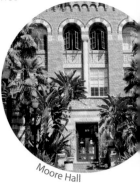

Take the time to explore the gardens at your leisure, or perhaps simply sit and relax in the green shade on one of the many benches. This oasis features plant life from all over the world, including many species of tropical and subtropical flora. The topography of UCLA's botanical gardens is a remnant of the ravine that used to

Moore Hall

run across the entire campus. Today, a water pump feeds the river that flows down the center of the gardens.

After spending some time in the gardens, exit back out onto Young Drive.

Turn right on Young Drive and retrace your steps along the perimeter of the campus. After crossing Westholme, you'll notice the barnlike structure of the Faculty Center on your right.

Just past Murphy Hall, turn right on Dickson Court (instead of continuing straight, which would take you back to the sculpture garden) on a path that will take you past the School of Law on your left.

Turn left to continue on Young Drive, following it all the way back to the intersection with Hilgard Avenue, where you began.

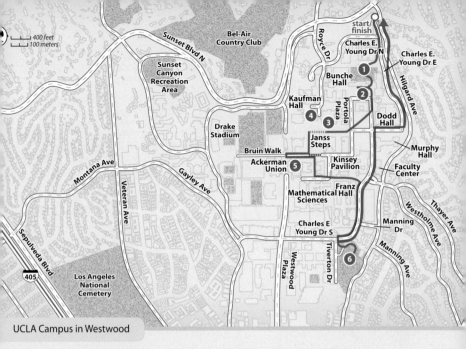

UCLA Campus in Westwood

Points of Interest

1 Franklin D. Murphy Sculpture Garden Charles E. Young Drive E., Los Angeles, CA 90095; 310-443-7000, tinyurl.com/murphysculpturegarden

2 Bunche Hall 11282 Portola Plaza, Los Angeles, CA 90095

3 Royce Hall 340 Royce Drive, Los Angeles, CA 90095; 310-825-2101, roycehall.org

4 Fowler Museum at UCLA 308 Charles E. Young Drive N., Los Angeles, CA 90024; 310-825-4361, fowler.ucla.edu

5 Ackerman Union/UCLA Store 308 Westwood Plaza, Los Angeles, CA 90095; 310-825-7711, asucla.edu/student-union

6 Mildred E. Mathias Botanical Garden 777 Tiverton Drive, Los Angeles, CA 90095; 310-825-1260, botgard.ucla.edu. Please call ahead to make sure the gardens are open at the time of your walk.

Helms Bakery made the official bread of the 1932 Olympics.

10 Central Culver City

BOUNDARIES: Venice Blvd., La Cienega Blvd., Baldwin Hills, Overland Ave.
DISTANCE: 3.5 miles
DIFFICULTY: Moderate
PARKING: Metered parking is available on Washington Blvd.
NEAREST METRO STATION: Expo Line (Culver City)

Culver City flew under the radar for a long time, playing the role of a fairly quiet residential suburb with a perfectly serviceable downtown district and a handful of decent restaurants. But how things have changed: downtown Culver City is now a thriving dining destination, and the excellent selection of eateries has spilled over into the historic Art Deco buildings of the old Helms Bakery complex. This walk takes in Culver City's hippest corridors, as well as one of the city's finest parks, which offers breathtaking views of the LA Basin on a clear day.

Walk Description

Start on Helms Avenue north of Washington Boulevard. This section of the street has been turned into a pedestrian-only plaza as part of the revitalization of the Helms Bakery District, a collection of great restaurants and upscale furniture stores housed in the 1930s-era Art Deco warehouse buildings of what used to be Helms Bakery. The large neon sign atop the structure has been restored and is now a famous local landmark, shining bright and colorful at night as it flashes the words HELMS OLYMPIC BREAD.

Turn right on Washington Boulevard. As you approach National Boulevard, you'll pass ❶ **Surfas Culinary District,** which stocks all manner of specialty and hard-to-find cooking supplies and ingredients and offers free cooking demos in the on-site test kitchen. In short, it's a foodie's dream come true. There's even an on-site café where you can grab a quick and tasty lunch or sweet, buttery pastry. And if you look across the street to the left, you'll notice an interesting mural of a girl in a colorful dress standing in front of a black-and-white creature holding flowers. Titled *The Guardian*, this artwork was a collaboration between street artists Bumblebee and Zio Ziegler.

Continue across National Boulevard, passing the Culver City Metro Expo Line station on your right. As you continue to head southwest on Washington, you'll pass a new creative office development on the left, its parking structure adorned with another colorful mural.

If you haven't already crossed to the other side of Washington Boulevard, do so at the intersection of Higuera Street. The Rapt Studio building on the corner features yet another colorful, eye-catching mural on the Higuera side of the building, this one by artist Jason Woodside.

Cross Higuera Street to continue on Washington, passing the white Art Deco buildings of Sony Pictures Animation on your left.

After crossing Ince Boulevard, keep straight. You'll pass ❷ **The Culver Studios;** the building facade resembles a grand Colonial mansion and will be instantly recognizable to film buffs from the opening credits of *Gone with the Wind*. Built by Thomas H. Ince in 1919, it has also been home to RKO, DeMille, and Desilu studios and continues to be a popular filming location today.

Continue straight ahead through the pedestrian plaza that is home to the ArcLight Cinemas, several restaurants, and ❸ **The Culver Hotel.** Another historic landmark, this establishment opened as the Hotel Hunt in 1924 to accommodate the many actors who filmed at The Culver Studios across the street. In fact, the Munchkins from *The Wizard of Oz* had such a good time here that they held a reunion of the surviving cast members at the hotel in 1997. The plaza also features a charming dancing lion statue and splash pad, popular with kids during the warm months.

After passing through the plaza, turn right to cross Culver Boulevard at Cardiff Avenue. After crossing, turn left, crossing Cardiff to head southwest on Culver Boulevard. This is the heart of the downtown Culver City dining district, and you'll pass several restaurants—all quite good—in quick succession, including ❹ **Tender Greens,** ❺ **Honey's Kettle,** and ❻ **Akasha.**

At Watseka Avenue, cross the street at the crosswalk on your left, and then continue across the second crosswalk to end up on the pleasant, jacaranda-shaded island between Washington and Culver Boulevards. Continue straight ahead, passing even more restaurants, as well as the ❼ **Kirk Douglas Theatre.** You'll see the massive Sony Pictures Studios complex directly ahead.

Turn left on Duquesne Avenue; City Hall is on the southeast corner. Take a quick detour through the courtyard to admire the brick fountains, and then continue southeast on Duquesne, passing the police station and a couple of blocks of mostly older houses and apartment buildings. Baldwin Hills lies straight ahead; you may see hikers and stair climbers along the left side of the ridge (see next walk).

After a couple of blocks, you will come to the pedestrian and bicycle entrance to the Ballona Creek bike path, which leads all the way to the beach. A useful map of the area stands near the gate, and on the wall alongside the entrance ramp is a community mural composed of colorful tiles, paintings, and mosaics that is well worth checking out. And you can't miss the giant metal sculpture of an urn on the other side of the waterway. Continue on Duquesne Avenue, crossing Jefferson Boulevard.

Continue walking on the sidewalk up the hill past the entrance to **8 Culver City Park.** To the right you'll see a creatively designed playground with lots of great climbing elements for kids, as well as a skate park.

When you see a parking lot on the other side of the street, cross at the crosswalk and then cut through the lot to the base of the zigzagging wooden ramp; follow the ramp uphill. This is the Culver City Park Interpretive Nature Trail, which gives way to a dirt path and passes a ropes challenge course before the wooden ramp resumes. As you continue your climb, take a moment to enjoy the view of Culver City below and see if you can spot the giant rainbow sculpture on the Sony Pictures lot.

More stellar vistas await once you reach the park at the top of the ramp, encompassing everything from the Pacific Ocean to downtown LA. *Homage to Ballona Creek,* an impressive sundial sculpture by artist Lucy Blake-Elahi, also graces the bluff.

Turn right from the top of the ramp to walk around the perimeter of the baseball field. Just after passing the restrooms, look for a set of four flights of stairs on your right, and descend. A couple of wells for the nearby Inglewood Oil Field pump away on the hill directly ahead.

Turn right at the bottom of the stairs to head downhill, passing a dog park on your left.

Turn right again at the stop sign to get back onto Duquesne, crossing at the crosswalk to return to the sidewalk. Retrace your steps back down the hill, once again crossing Jefferson Boulevard.

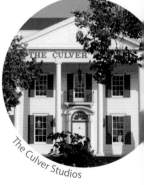

The Culver Studios

Turn right on Lucerne after crossing Ballona Creek; you'll follow this quiet residential street for several blocks.

Turn left on Higuera Street, which is lined with exceptionally cute and well-maintained homes. At the corner of Poinsettia Court, you'll notice Jerry's Market, your quintessential neighborhood bodega. After passing the Citydog! Club boarding and doggy day care facility on your right, you'll spot the Rapt Studio mural from earlier in the walk.

Turn right on Washington Boulevard to retrace your steps back toward the Helms Bakery District.

Return to the starting point of your walk, at the corner of Helms Avenue and Washington Boulevard.

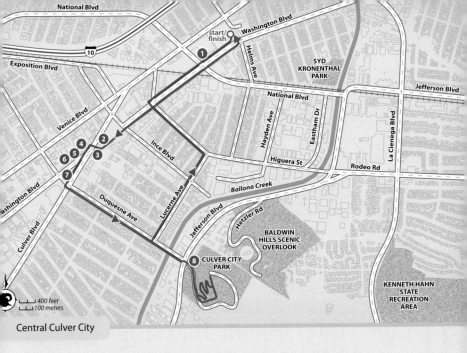

Central Culver City

Points of Interest

1 **Surfas Culinary District** 8777 Washington Blvd., Culver City, CA 90232; 310-559-4770, surfasonline.com

2 **The Culver Studios** 9336 Washington Blvd., Culver City, CA 90232; 310-202-1234, theculverstudios.com

3 **The Culver Hotel** 9400 Culver Blvd., Culver City, CA 90232; 310-558-9400, culverhotel.com

4 **Tender Greens** 9523 Culver Blvd., Culver City, CA 90232; 310-842-8300, tinyurl.com/tendergreenscc

5 **Honey's Kettle** 9537 Culver Blvd., Culver City, CA 90232; 310-202-5453, honeyskettle.com

6 **Akasha** 9543 Culver Blvd., Culver City, CA 90232; 310-845-1700, akasharestaurant.com

7 **Kirk Douglas Theatre** 9820 Washington Blvd., Culver City, CA 90232; 213-628-2772, centertheatregroup.org/visit/kirk-douglas-theatre

8 **Culver City Park** 9910 Jefferson Blvd., Culver City, CA 90232

Panoramic views from the Baldwin Hills stairs

11 Culver City's Baldwin Hills Stairs and Hayden Tract

BOUNDARIES: La Cienega Blvd., National Blvd., Washington Blvd., Duquesne Ave.
DISTANCE: About 3.5 miles
DIFFICULTY: Strenuous (includes stairways)
PARKING: Free street parking is available on Jefferson Blvd.
NEAREST METRO STATION: Expo Line (Jefferson/La Cienega)

Constructed in 2006, the stairs leading up to the Baldwin Hills Scenic Overlook are so mammoth that they can reportedly be seen from space. They also represent an epic opportunity to get outdoors and work up a sweat right in the middle of our big sprawling, concrete-bound metropolis; plus, they're totally free and accessible to everyone.

The straight-up shot of 282 steps leading to the viewing platform is challenging, to say the least: the steps are giant and uneven, and many are much taller than typical stairs. But the 360-degree views of Los Angeles at the top are positively killer—and worth the killer workout.

Directly north of the stairway lies the Hayden Tract. This formerly run-down industrial neighborhood underwent a transformation beginning in the 1980s, when developers Frederick and Laurie Samitaur Smith partnered with architect Eric Owen Moss to convert industrial warehouses into striking contemporary creative and office spaces.

Walk Description

Begin at the intersection of Hetzler Road and Jefferson Boulevard. Look for the big sign reading TRAILHEAD, and follow the dirt path up the hill until you reach the base of the stairs.

Climb the 282 stairs to reach the ❶ **Baldwin Hills Scenic Overlook.** Wander around the viewing platform and trails at the top of the 511-foot peak to soak in the awesome panoramic views of the greater Los Angeles area.

Follow the path to the right around the viewing platform to continue to the gracefully designed, glass-walled visitor center. Because of budget cutbacks, the center is open only occasionally, but the public restrooms are accessible to hikers.

Retrace your steps from the visitor center back to the top of the stairs, and descend the first set until you reach the point where the stairway crosses the dirt path.

Turn left on the path to follow it as it zigzags all the way to the bottom of the hill, crossing back and forth across the stairs. You will come across a couple of forks in the path, but as long as you stay on the dirt and continue downhill, you'll end up in the right place. Taking the trail down, as opposed to the stairs, is much easier on the knees and offers the chance to slow down and enjoy the sights and scents of native plants, critters, and insects without fear of being trampled by an overzealous climber.

When you return to the trailhead, turn right on Jefferson. This industrial stretch is not very pleasant or attractive, but there are some interesting plant and garden stores along the way. After just under a third of a mile, bear left at the split in the road to stay on Jefferson.

Make a quick left onto Higuera Street. (The street sign says RODEO ROAD heading to the right.) You'll see a sign welcoming you to the Hayden Tract, and then you'll pass the LA School of Gymnastics on your left.

Turn right on Hayden Avenue. Here, the architectural style clearly shifts from industrial/commercial to industrial chic. The next three blocks are home to advertising and design firms, dance studios, and other types of creative enterprises. At 3585, you'll want to leave the sidewalk to take a closer look at the elevated cactus garden designed by Eric Owen Moss.

As you approach National Boulevard, you'll come to the ❷ **Conjunctive Points** complex on your right. This offbeat and striking architectural landmark comprises the intimidating angular black Stealth building as well as the topsy-turvy Samitaur Tower at the corner of Hayden and National. If the parking-lot security guard gives you the go-ahead, continue into the complex to see more innovative structures and designs.

Turn right at the corner of Hayden and National, and walk one block to Eastham Drive. Directly across National Boulevard, in ❸ **Syd Kronenthal Park** is an entrance to the Ballona Creek Bike Path. The next exit point is a little over a mile south down the path at Duquesne Avenue, or one could take it all the way to the ocean—something to keep in mind if you return on two wheels. But today you're walking, so turn right on Eastham.

The buildings on Eastham reflect the converted industrial sensibility of their neighbors on Hayden. Continue back to Higuera and turn left.

From here, you'll retrace your steps back to your starting point: turn right on Jefferson, and follow the road as it curves to the right and leads back to the corner of Hetzler Road.

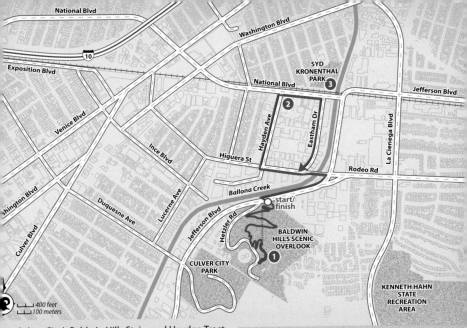

Culver City's Baldwin Hills Stairs and Hayden Tract

Points of Interest

1. **Baldwin Hills Scenic Overlook** 6300 Hetzler Road, Culver City, CA 90232

2. **Conjunctive Points** Hayden Avenue between Higuera Street and National Boulevard, Culver City, CA 90232

3. **Syd Kronenthal Park** 3459 McManus Ave., Culver City, CA 90232

12 West Hollywood Design District

BOUNDARIES: Melrose Ave., San Vicente Blvd., Santa Monica Blvd., Kings Rd.
DISTANCE: About 2.25 miles
DIFFICULTY: Easy
PARKING: Free street parking is available on Kings Rd.

This tour of the best West Hollywood has to offer begins at the Schindler House, an early-modern architectural gem and home of the MAK Center for Art and Architecture. The walk then goes on to explore the *très chic* stretch of Melrose Avenue and its offshoot, Melrose Place, which are home to high-end home-furnishings galleries and couture boutiques.

Easily the most dramatic destination on this journey is the Pacific Design Center, a colossal collection of blue, green, and red glass buildings that house more than a hundred interior design showrooms.

Walk Description

Begin on Kings Road, just south of Willoughby Avenue. The ❶ **Schindler House** sits at 835 Kings Road, hidden from view by a tall bamboo hedge. If it's open at the time of your walk, proceed along the dirt path to the MAK Center office and bookstore, where you can submit a donation before exploring. The Schindler House is a building like no other. Composed of unadorned concrete and dark-stained wood, the one-story structure manages to feel airy and light despite the low, wood-beamed ceilings. Furnishings are modern and sparse, and a couple of rooms feature copper-topped fireplaces. The indoor and outdoor spaces are seamlessly integrated; clear plastic curtains separate the rooms of the house from the peaceful green gardens, which are shrouded from the surrounding area by more bamboo.

After leaving the Schindler House, continue south on Kings Road toward Melrose Avenue. Next door to the Schindler House is an apartment complex called Habitat 825. The sleek, neomodern structure, designed by Lorcan O'Herlihy, has received some flack for the way it towers over the south side of Schindler's famed creation, although the architect did make an effort to respect his neighbor when designing the building.

Turn right on Melrose. Across the street is ❷ **Mel & Rose,** a wine-and-spirits store that's distinguished by a delightfully tacky giant wine bottle with a neon sign.

Bear slightly right at the fork in the road to make your way onto Melrose Place. This pleasantly landscaped street is home to a collection of expensive clothing labels and interior design showrooms.

Turn left on La Cienega Boulevard, and walk to the intersection of Melrose Avenue and La Cienega.

Cross La Cienega Boulevard. On the southwest corner of La Cienega and Melrose is a singularly ugly strip mall composed of black-and-white horizontally striped marble.

At 8565 Melrose is ❸ **Urth Caffé,** an invariably crowded café that caters to people who want to indulge in rich foods made with guilt-free ingredients. ❹ **Le Pain Quotidien,** in the next block, is a slightly more low-key option, with a pleasant wraparound porch for outdoor dining.

At 8687 Melrose Ave., just before San Vicente Boulevard, you finally arrive at the ❺ **Pacific Design Center.** Up close, the massive blue-glass structure is striking—

and almost intimidating. At night, the effect is even more dramatic, as the tall, pod-shaped spotlights bathe the building's exterior in a red glow. The design center is home to 130 showrooms displaying furnishings from an array of designers and manufacturers, ranging in style from traditional to contemporary. The center also frequently hosts exhibitions, lectures, and special events. The Museum of Contemporary Art (MOCA) even has a satellite gallery here.

The main entrance to the center is located around the corner on San Vicente. You'll pass a giant metal sculpture of a chair as you turn the corner. The entryway is situated off a large, open courtyard, which is dominated by a spectacular dancing fountain. Call ahead or visit pacificdesigncenter.com to see if there is an interesting exhibit either at MOCA or in the design center at the time of your visit. The **6** **West Hollywood Library,** across the street at 625 N. San Vicente Blvd., is worth a visit for its clean, pleasant, and light-filled interior design. Next door, at 647 N. San Vicente, you'll notice West Hollywood Park, which features a playground, public swimming pool, and tennis courts.

Cut across through the fountain plaza of the Design Center, and then head up the stairs next to the red building (the most recent addition to the complex). Continue north on San Vicente, passing the sheriff's station on your right at the corner of Santa Monica Boulevard.

Turn right on Santa Monica. You're now in the heart of historically gay West Holly-wood, which remains a nighttime hot spot for the LGBT community with its restaurants, bars, and clubs. To the north, you can spot the hotels and oversize billboards of the Sunset Strip.

Continue east along Santa Monica to the intersection of Hancock Avenue, cross-ing Santa Monica Boulevard at the crosswalk to head north on this side street.

Head uphill on Hancock for one block and then make a right onto West Knoll Drive, a relatively quiet street of pleasant-looking houses and apartment buildings. When you come to the small roundabout adorned with a colorful tiled pillar, continue straight ahead on West Knoll.

After a short distance, West Knoll Drive reconnects you with Santa Monica Boulevard.

Across the street, at 8520 Santa Monica Blvd., is California's first outpost of the insanely popular New York City burger joint **7 Shake Shack.**

Turn left on Santa Monica, walk to the intersection of La Cienega Boulevard, and then cross to the east side of the street.

Turn right on La Cienega and then take an immediate left on Romaine Street. You've now left the hustle and bustle of the boulevard and entered a quiet residential neighborhood.

After four blocks, Romaine Street ends at **8 Kings Road Park,** a dog-friendly haven tucked between two apartment buildings. The shady little park features a small playground, benches arranged around a burbling fountain, and public restrooms, as well as dog-waste bags to ensure that owners clean up after their pooches.

After visiting the park, head south on Kings Road toward your starting point. The street is lined with courtyard apartment buildings; the "Tree House," a narrow, dark-shingled complex at 906 N. Kings Road, stands out from the rest.

Cross Willoughby Avenue to return to your starting point near the Schindler House, at 835 Kings Road.

Designer Name: Rudolf M. Schindler

Rudolf M. Schindler was an Austrian-born architect who was inspired by Frank Lloyd Wright. After he began working for Wright in Chicago in 1918, his mentor sent him to Los Angeles to supervise the construction of the Hollyhock House (see Walk 20, Los Feliz). It was here that Schindler established himself as an innovative and progressive architect in his own right. In 1922, he created West Hollywood's Kings Road House (now commonly referred to as the Schindler House), a building that is considered an icon of early modern architecture. The minimalist structure is an example of what Schindler described as "space architecture." It functioned as his home and studio until he died in 1953. The house communicates a singular blend of old and new; while the building design is undoubtedly modern, the low ceilings and organic, unadorned materials reveal the influence of indigenous architecture.

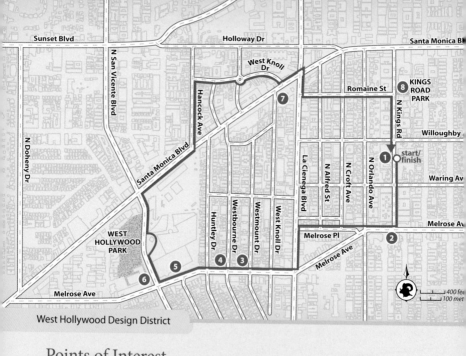

West Hollywood Design District

Points of Interest

1 Schindler House/MAK Center for Art and Architecture 835 N. Kings Road, West Hollywood, CA 90069; 323-651-1510, makcenter.org

2 Mel & Rose 8344 Melrose Ave., West Hollywood, CA 90069; 323-655-5557, melandrose.com

3 Urth Caffé 8565 Melrose Ave., West Hollywood, CA 90069; 310-659-0628, urthcaffe.com

4 Le Pain Quotidien 8607 Melrose Ave., West Hollywood, CA 90069; 310-854-3700, lepainquotidien.com/store/melrose

5 Pacific Design Center and MOCA 8687 Melrose Ave., West Hollywood, CA 90069; 310-657-0800, pacificdesigncenter.com

6 West Hollywood Library 625 N. San Vicente Blvd., West Hollywood, CA 90069; 310-652-5340, colapublib.org/libs/whollywood

7 Shake Shack 8520 Santa Monica Blvd., West Hollywood, CA 90069; 323-488-3010, shakeshack.com/location/west-hollywood

8 Kings Road Park 1000 N. Kings Road, West Hollywood, CA 90069

Tragic tableau at the La Brea Tar Pits

13 Miracle Mile

BOUNDARIES: Wilshire Blvd., Fairfax Ave., Beverly Blvd., Martel Ave./Hauser Blvd.
DISTANCE: About 2.5 miles
DIFFICULTY: Easy
PARKING: Free parking is available on the north side of Sixth Street. Metered parking is available on the south side.

The Miracle Mile district is a prized area in Los Angeles, in large part because of its proximity to just about anyplace you might want to go. This neighborhood is home to the Los Angeles County Museum of Art (LACMA), the historic Farmers Market, and—unlikely as it may seem in the middle of this bustling city—one of the world's most famous fossil sites. The La Brea Tar Pits, adjacent to LACMA, are said to have the largest and most diverse collection of animal and plant fossils from the Ice Age, tens of thousands of years ago. After exploring the tar pits and fossil excavation sites, you'll get a strong dose of modern-day Los Angeles at The Grove, an enormously popular outdoor mall created by mega-developer Rick Caruso that brings to mind Disneyland's Main Street, U.S.A.

Walk Description

Begin at the corner of Sixth Street and Curson Avenue, and head south on Curson toward Wilshire Boulevard.

Just before you reach Wilshire, you'll see an entrance to Hancock Park on your right. Not to be confused with the upscale neighborhood, the park is home to the ❶ La Brea Tar Pits and Museum, which oversees the preservation, study, excavation, and cleaning of fossils from the pits. The ❷ Los Angeles County Museum of Art (LACMA) is also here.

Enter Hancock Park (there are public restrooms near the entrance), and notice the La Brea Tar Pits Museum on your right. Take a few minutes to follow the steps to the roof of the building, and you'll be rewarded with a view over the museum's lush tropical garden and koi pond. It's peaceful up here, with the sound of a trickling waterfall and birds flitting in and out of the oasis below. The garden is topped

Back Story: La Brea Tar Pits

The La Brea Tar Pits Museum (formerly the Page Museum), on the site of a 19th-century Mexican land grant called Rancho La Brea, gives visitors a taste of Los Angeles as it was 10,000–40,000 years ago, during the final Ice Age of the Pleistocene epoch. The source of the asphalt pits that serve as the museum's excavation sites is a large underground petroleum reservoir located a short distance north of the park.

This extraordinarily sticky piece of land was the site of roughly 10,000 creatures' demise over the span of 30,000 years. The unlucky victims included small and large mammals, birds, and insects (but no dinosaurs, which had long since gone extinct during the Pleistocene). After an animal, such as a saber-toothed cat or dire wolf, became stuck in the goo, it would fall prey to carnivorous mammals and birds, some of which would themselves get caught in the mire. Today, the resulting collection of Ice Age fossils is one of the largest and most diverse in the world.

with an intricate, open ironwork cage of sorts, the sides of which are decorated with a bas-relief of prehistoric creatures.

Return to ground level and walk south across the park to observe the largest of the tar pits, where the smell of liquid asphalt is reminiscent of hot days on the playground. The museum has erected a heartbreaking sculptural tableau of a baby mammoth accompanied, presumably, by its father on the shore of the pond; the baby is wailing in sadness as it watches its mother get sucked into the muck. You can still see evidence of geologic activity on these grounds, with the occasional bubbling up of gases through the water's murky surface.

Head west through the park, away from Curson. Hancock Park is a popular place for locals to walk their dogs, play Frisbee, or simply stroll across the hilly green lawns. You'll pass the Pavilion for Japanese Art on your left; this building, with its swooping architectural style, is part of LACMA. Continue through the park, passing a fossil excavation site on your right and the LACMA complex on your left. Soon you reach the entry pavilion for the Broad Contemporary Art Museum at LACMA. This boxy travertine structure, designed by Renzo Piano and opened in 2008, was built with a $60 million gift from philanthropists Eli and Edythe Broad, who also funded The Broad museum in downtown LA (see Walk 30).

Turn right opposite the entry pavilion to exit the park.

Turn left on Sixth Street.

Walk one block to Fairfax Avenue, turn right, and continue about half a mile. On your right you'll pass the western side of the massive Park La Brea apartment complex, whose Colonial Revival multifamily units were constructed in 1944. On your left you'll pass ❸ **Molly Malone's Irish Pub,** at 575 Fairfax. And you won't miss the four-story Art Deco building that's home to ❹ **Samy's Camera** at 431 Fairfax.

Cross Third Street and enter the ❺ **Farmers Market,** right next to the sign that reads MEET ME AT THIRD AND FAIRFAX.

Walk into the market through the entrance near Du-par's restaurant, and make your way through the maze of food stands, coffee shops, butchers, bakeries, produce counters, and souvenir shops at this popular spot. Needless to say, this is a great place to grab a bite. Notable eateries include Loteria, a Mexico City–style taco stand; the Gumbo Pot for Cajun food; the Pampas Grill Brazilian *churrascaria;* and the Banana Leaf for Singaporean food. As you make your way through the market, head toward the northeast corner, where you will exit straight into ❻ **The Grove** shopping center.

Finding your way through The Grove is easy, as it's pretty much laid out in a straight line. It might not be so easy to make it through without blowing your paycheck, however. Most of the stores here are upscale, and there are several nice restaurants, a huge movie theater, an Apple Store, and a three-story Barnes & Noble.

The Grove distinguishes itself from Southern California's other outdoor malls with an old-fashioned trolley and a large fountain shooting streams of water that "dance" to the tunes of old standards by crooners such as Dean Martin and Frank Sinatra. It all makes for quite a spectacle, and it draws people in droves.

After passing Gap, turn left to exit the mall through the valet parking area onto The Grove Drive, and turn left.

On your right is ❼ **Pan Pacific Park.** This sunken expanse of rolling green lawns, playgrounds, playing fields, and jogging paths is relatively hidden from view of the surrounding streets, making it a delightful discovery if you're new to the area. Take some time to explore the park, which is usually filled with picnicking families and young athletes.

Continue north on The Grove Drive to the corner of Beverly Boulevard. On the southwest corner is ❽ **Erewhon,** one of LA's most established health food markets, offering any sort of vegetarian, vegan, organic, Kosher, macrobiotic, herbal, or gluten-free delicacy you could desire. It also features a juice bar and an extensive prepared-foods counter. If you've managed to hold out this long without stopping at one of the many eateries on this walk, you may want to pick up a wrap or salad to take on a picnic in the park across the street.

Back Story: Miracle Mile's Auspicious Beginning

The ironic thing about the Miracle Mile is that it's not miraculous. The stretch of Wilshire Boulevard between La Brea Avenue and Fairfax Avenue is vibrant and pleasant, to be sure, with a distinctive mix of cultural institutions, tall office buildings, and charming residential neighborhoods, but it's no grander than LA's other affluent districts. In the early 1920s, however, it was a dusty 18-acre expanse of farmland. Developer A. W. Ross got the idea to transform it into a prestigious shopping and business district, and to this day, many of the original commercial buildings along Wilshire bustle with corporate activity: a dream come true for Ross, whose original designation—Miracle Mile—stuck.

Turn right on Beverly Boulevard, passing the post office on the south side of the street before coming to the **Pan Pacific Park Recreation Center,** (see ❼), which is constructed of red- and green-painted bricks in the distinctive Streamline Moderne style.

Turn right on Vista Street to enter the Historic Preservation Overlay Zone (HPOZ), known as Miracle Mile North. (An HPOZ is an area that the city of Los Angeles has determined to have historic, architectural, aesthetic, or cultural significance.) Continue along Vista for one block, noticing the various residential architectural styles. The modest-sized homes are beautifully maintained, their preservation carefully overseen by the HPOZ board. The predominant styles are Spanish Colonial Revival, Tudor Revival, and American Colonial Revival.

Turn left on First Street and note the striking Norman cottage on the southeast corner of the street.

After one short block, turn right on Martel Avenue. Here you'll spot a classic example of the American Colonial Revival architectural style on the southeast corner, at 100 S. Martel. Continue south on Martel. After you cross Second Street, notice the collection of distinctive Spanish duplexes on your right, from 187 to 217 S. Martel.

The congruity of layout and the intricate wrought-iron details suggest that these buildings were all designed by the same talented architect.

Cross Third Street. At this point, Martel Avenue becomes Hauser Boulevard. Continue on Hauser for several blocks through the Park La Brea apartment complex. The distinctive 13-story towers of Park La Brea were built in 1950 in response to the post–World War II housing shortage. On your left, look for the relatively new, Italian-influenced Palazzo division of the complex.

Turn right on Sixth Street, and then cross Curson to return to the start of your walk.

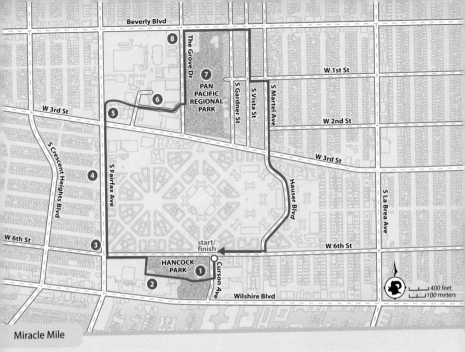

Miracle Mile

Points of Interest

1. **La Brea Tar Pits and Museum/Hancock Park** 5801 Wilshire Blvd., Los Angeles, CA 90036; 323-934-7243, tarpits.org

2. **Los Angeles County Museum of Art** 5905 Wilshire Blvd., Los Angeles, CA 90036; 323-857-6000, lacma.org

3. **Molly Malone's Irish Pub** 575 S. Fairfax Ave., Los Angeles, CA 90036; 323-935-1577, mollymalonesla.com

4. **Samy's Camera** 431 S. Fairfax Ave., Los Angeles, CA 90036; 323-938-2420, samys.com

5. **Farmers Market** 6333 W. Third St., Los Angeles, CA 90036; 323-933-9211, farmersmarketla.com

6. **The Grove** 189 The Grove Drive, Los Angeles, CA 90036; 888-315-8883, thegrovela.com

7. **Pan Pacific Park and Recreation Center** 7600 Beverly Blvd., Los Angeles, CA 90036; 323-939-8874, laparks.org/reccenter/pan-pacific

8. **Erewhon** 7660 Beverly Blvd., Los Angeles, CA 90036; 323-937-0777, erewhonmarket.com

Margaret Herrick Library, Academy of Motion Picture Arts and Sciences

14 Carthay Circle and South Carthay

BOUNDARIES: La Cienega Blvd., Wilshire Blvd., Fairfax Ave., Whitworth Dr.
DISTANCE: About 2 miles
DIFFICULTY: Easy
PARKING: Metered parking is available on La Cienega Blvd. and Gregory Way.

This walk explores the neighborhoods of Carthay Circle and South Carthay in the bustling Miracle Mile district, just southeast of Beverly Hills. Although they're right next to each other, these two neighborhoods—whose houses and apartment buildings have distinct architectural integrity and cohesiveness—have been designated as separate Historic Preservation Overlay Zones by the city of Los Angeles.

Carthay Circle is composed primarily of Spanish Colonial Revival–style homes, with a few Tudor Revival and American Colonial Revival houses. The architecture in South Carthay is a little more cohesive, consisting almost entirely of Spanish Colonial Revivals. Both neighborhoods are well maintained and relatively isolated from the busy surrounding boulevards, making this a peaceful oasis in the middle of one of LA's thriving business districts.

Walk Description

The first part of this walk covers Carthay Circle, which features a mix of single-family homes and duplexes in an appealing variety of architectural styles, ranging from Spanish Colonial Revival to Tudor. Begin at La Cienega Park, on the east side of La Cienega Boulevard at the corner of Gregory Way. Head east on Gregory along the northern border of the park.

Turn right on Schumacher Drive. At 865 Schumacher is an interesting stone house with a crenellated roofline that gives it the incongruous look of a medieval castle.

Turn left on Moore Drive. Notice the pair of Spanish-style homes on the northeast and southeast corners, each of which is dominated by a squat towerlike structure.

After less than a block, turn left on Santa Ynez Way, a narrow sidewalk alley bordered by a hedge.

Santa Ynez emerges onto Hayes Drive. Turn right and continue about a block.

After crossing Foster Drive, you'll find yourself on a street named Commodore Sloat Drive.

Look for ❶ **Carthay Circle Park,** a narrow greenway between two office buildings, on your left. (Another small parklet on your right features a large boulder with a plaque memorializing a mail-carrying pioneer by the name of Snowshoe Thompson.) Turn left to cut through to San Vicente Boulevard. At the end of the greenway, facing San Vicente, notice the sculpture of Juan Bautista de Anza, who led the first settlers from Sonora, Mexico, to California.

Turn right on San Vicente Boulevard, cross Carrillo Drive, and then take the crosswalk across San Vicente.

Continue straight on the street that is now called McCarthy Vista for two short blocks to Wilshire Boulevard.

Turn left to head west on Wilshire. The museums of the Miracle Mile district are just a couple of blocks to the east.

At La Jolla Avenue, you'll see an alley cutting between two tall office buildings on your left; turn here. This drab alley turns into Capistrano Way, a peaceful sidewalk trimmed with bougainvillea, ficus, and fruit trees.

As you emerge from Capistrano Way, turn right on Warner Drive.

Warner ends at San Vicente Boulevard. Carefully cross San Vicente; a grassy island dividing this busy street makes it a little easier to cross even though there is no crosswalk.

Once across San Vicente, you'll see a sign for San Gabriel Way a short distance southeast (to your left); this is yet another sidewalk alley. Turn right to follow San Gabriel Way through to Commodore Sloat Drive. Notice the American Colonial Revival house opposite the alley at 6440 Commodore Sloat.

Turn left on Commodore Sloat and walk about two blocks, briefly retracing your steps from earlier in the walk.

Turn right on Carrillo Drive. Carthay Center Elementary School is on your right.

When you reach the intersection with Olympic Boulevard, cross the street using the crosswalk in front of the entrance to the school. (There is also an underground tunnel for traversing the busy boulevard, but it isn't always unlocked.)

Now you are in the neighborhood of South Carthay. Continue straight on what is now Crescent Heights Boulevard. This block is distinguished by gorgeous, immaculately maintained, Spanish-style duplexes and small apartment buildings.

Turn right on Whitworth Drive and continue two blocks to La Jolla Avenue.

Turn right on La Jolla. Here the residences are primarily one-story, single-family homes. The predominant architectural style is Spanish Colonial Revival, identified by its low-pitched, red-tile roofs and arched doorways and windows. Notice that many of these Spanish Colonial houses feature stained-glass details in the windows, just one example of the many decorative accents that distinguish this timelessly elegant architectural style. It is obvious why the city chose to designate this as a protected architectural district.

Turn left on Olympic Place, which is prettily lined with magnolia trees, and continue one block to Orlando Avenue.

Turn right on Orlando and walk one block to Olympic Boulevard.

Turn left on Olympic. On the south side of Olympic, you'll notice several apartment buildings in the châteaulike French Normandy style, which stand out from the other residences in the area.

Turn right on La Cienega Boulevard. You'll pass the distinctive shield-shaped BEVERLY HILLS sign, letting you know you have entered its glamorous city limits. On your left you'll pass the impressive Spanish Colonial–style **❷ Margaret Herrick Library of the Academy of Motion Picture Arts and Sciences.**

Return to your starting point near the intersection of La Cienega and Gregory Way.

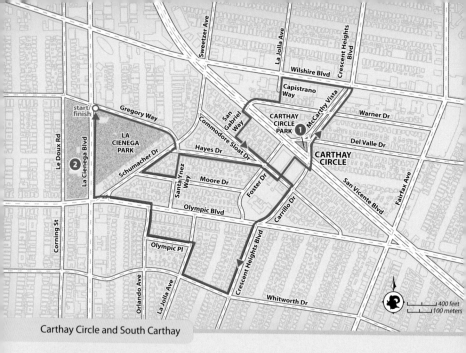

Carthay Circle and South Carthay

Points of Interest

1. **Carthay Circle Park** Commodore Sloat Drive north to Wilshire Boulevard, Los Angeles, CA 90048

2. **Margaret Herrick Library, Academy of Motion Picture Arts and Sciences** 333 S. La Cienega Blvd., Beverly Hills, CA 90211; 310-247-3020, oscars.org/library

The imposing Art Deco entrance to the Hollywood Bowl

15 Hollywood's High Tower and Whitley Heights

BOUNDARIES: US 101, Outpost Dr., Franklin Ave., Cahuenga Blvd.
DISTANCE: About 3 miles
DIFFICULTY: Moderate (includes stairways)
PARKING: Street parking is available on Camrose Dr. (pay attention to posted signs), and there's also a parking lot for visitors to the Hollywood Heritage Museum, just north of Milner on Highland Ave. Please be aware that parking anywhere in this vicinity on summer evenings can be dicey because of Hollywood Bowl parking restrictions.
NEAREST METRO STATION: Red Line (Hollywood Blvd. and Highland Ave.)

Tucked between the Hollywood Bowl and Camrose Drive in the Hollywood Hills sits the cozy and unusual High Tower neighborhood, which feels like an exciting peek into old Hollywood. The homes along Alta Loma Terrace, the pedestrian pathway at the top of the hill, are accessible either by stairs or by the Bolognese-style "high tower" elevator at the northern end of High Tower Drive. The Carl Kay–designed duplex immediately adjacent to the tower was featured as Philip Marlowe's apartment in the 1973 classic *The Long Goodbye*.

After a quick detour to the adjacent Hollywood Bowl complex, this route crosses Highland Avenue to explore Whitley Heights. Most of the homes in this neighborhood were built between 1918 and 1928, and the predominant architectural style is Spanish Colonial Revival. The seclusion and beauty of the area attracted such stars as Rudolph Valentino, Judy Garland, and Charlie Chaplin during Hollywood's heyday. Alas, the construction of US 101 in 1946–47 divided the hill in two, demolishing 40 historic homes in the process. To maintain what's left, the Historic Preservation Overlay Zone alliance has granted the neighborhood protected status. Today, Whitley Heights is still home to entertainment-industry professionals, and many of the original Mediterranean homes are as lovely as ever, but the address doesn't hold the same prestige it once did.

Walk Description

Begin at the northwest corner of Highland Avenue and Camrose Drive near Highland Camrose Park, a quiet sanctuary walled off from Highland Avenue that provides a convenient picnic area for patrons of the nearby Hollywood Bowl. Head away from Highland to go west on Camrose.

Turn right on Rockledge Road. Straight ahead on Rockledge, you'll see a gorgeous Spanish-style home with extensive blue tile work and a long balcony of arches overlooking the front courtyard.

Follow the road as it curves up the hill. The Mediterranean houses are increasingly ornate and colorful as you continue upward; some even have castlelike architectural flourishes.

When you reach the end of the cul-de-sac, you'll come to Los Altos Place, a pedestrian walkway. Descend the short flight of stairs and continue along the narrow path between homes.

Cross High Tower Drive, which is lined with single-car garages for residents of the neighborhood's hilltop homes. To the right you'll see the pretty tower for which the street is named. This structure houses a locked elevator to which only residents have a key. Continue along the path on the other side of High Tower Drive.

Turn right on Broadview Terrace, another pedestrian path, and continue up the stairs. As you approach the tower, you'll notice a raised clearing on your right. This patch of land provides a nice vantage point from which to admire the southeast view of Hollywood.

Ascend the stairs next to High Tower.

Turn right on Alta Loma Terrace. This path is shady and peaceful, and the houses on either side are accessible only by way of this pathway; hence the detached rows of garages on the street below. Architectural styles range from Mediterranean to Japanese to rambling clapboard farmhouse.

Turn right to continue along Alta Loma Terrace. You'll come to a charming fairy-tale house with miniature doors and windows at 6840.

Turn left to descend the stairs.

At the bottom of the stairs you'll find yourself in a private, fenced-off parking lot for the residents of Alta Loma Terrace. Turn left to head toward the black iron gate exiting onto Highland Avenue.

On the other side of the gate, turn left on Highland and walk toward the parking lot for the ❶ **Hollywood Bowl.** Follow the sidewalk adjacent to the lot until you reach the main entrance to the Bowl, which is marked by the 1940 George Stanley Fountain, a beautiful Art Deco piece representing the muse of music.

Turn left to follow the pathway identified as Peppertree Lane uphill to the amphitheater. On your left is the Hollywood Bowl Museum. It's worth stopping in to see blown-up panoramic photos of the outdoor theater taken when it was first incorporated into its natural canyon surroundings in 1922, and to admire exhibits about the many legendary performers who have played here over the decades.

Eventually you arrive at a circular plaza surrounded by snack bars, the box office, and the Hollywood Bowl gift shop. If a concert is in session and you don't have tickets, you won't be able to explore much more. Otherwise, continue up the hill through the turnstiles and enter the massive outdoor venue, which seats nearly

18,000 people. If you're lucky, you might even be able to catch an artist in the middle of sound check. A summer evening at the Bowl is a quintessential LA experience that every resident should try to enjoy at least once a year.

To leave the Hollywood Bowl complex, return to the plaza in front of the box office and follow the signs for the Odin Path, which takes you along a walkway that runs behind the museum and eventually deposits you in the massive parking lot.

Turn left to cut through the parking lot back to Highland Avenue.

At Highland, turn right and follow the sidewalk back toward Highland Camrose Park.

When you return to the corner of Camrose and Highland, cross to the east side of Highland Avenue. At this point, the street name changes from Camrose to Milner Road. A park with shady picnic areas for Hollywood Bowl patrons, as well as the ❷ Hollywood Heritage Museum (open weekend afternoons only), is on your left. Pass the Whitley Terrace Steps next door to 6776 Milner—you'll descend these later—and follow the road as it curves left, past romantic Mediterranean houses built up against the hill on your right. There are charming, cottagelike homes on your left. A posted sign indicates that you've entered the Whitley Heights Historical Preservation Overlay Zone.

The aptly named High Tower

Continue uphill and bear right to stay on Milner at the split in the road; you'll notice a stunning Spanish home on the corner with dark-stained wood and a huge, arched picture window. Two more Spanish Colonial Revival homes catch the eye at 6708 and 6718 Milner; both have a slightly imposing old-world beauty.

Turn right on Whitley Terrace. Several more elegant Spanish-style homes adorn the hill on your right. Many of the newer homes in Whitley Heights maintain the Spanish Colonial Revival style, integrating nicely into the old neighborhood. As Whitley Terrace curves left, note an interesting castlelike home at 6697 with unique floral tile murals and stained glass.

Ascend the wooden staircase on your left, just past 6681 Whitley Terrace—keep an eye out for it, as it can be easy to miss. A row of standalone garages lines the other side of the steps; most of Whitley Heights' homes were built in the 1920s with single-car garages, so the row garages were built to accommodate extra vehicles.

Turn left at the top of the steps onto Grace Avenue. You're now approaching the uppermost portion of Whitley Heights, where the homes have a peaceful, secluded quality. As you approach the top of the hill, you get a lovely view of Griffith Observatory in the distance. Note the gated road off to your left, at the point where Grace Avenue turns right—this is Kendra Court, the only street in the neighborhood that's closed to the public. Continue to follow Grace down the hill.

Turn right on Whitley Terrace. A couple of the houses on the left side of the street are modern in design, but most maintain the Mediterranean theme. While the homes on this side of the street appear to be on the small side compared with the stately homes on your right, they are actually quite grand, spilling down the hill on the other side and affording spectacular views of Hollywood and beyond.

Look for the sign for the staircase on your left that reads 2000 N. WHITLEY TERRACE STEPS (just past 6666 Whitley Terrace). There is a black wrought-iron gate at the top of the stairs, but it always seems to be unlocked. Descend the long staircase past several homes, a couple of which are accessible only by the stairs, lending them an appealing sense of being secret hideaways. As you head down, admire the charming vista of the hills on the other side of Highland; the red-tile roofs scattered among the treetops give the impression that you're in a seaside Mediterranean village thousands of miles away.

You'll encounter another gate at the bottom of the stairway, but, like the gate at the top, it should be unlocked. (In the unlikely case that either gate is locked, you can continue north/northeast on Whitley Terrace, turn left on Milner Road, and follow the street downhill to your starting point.)

At the bottom of the steps, turn left on Milner Road, and cross Highland Avenue to return to where you began near the corner of Highland and Camrose.

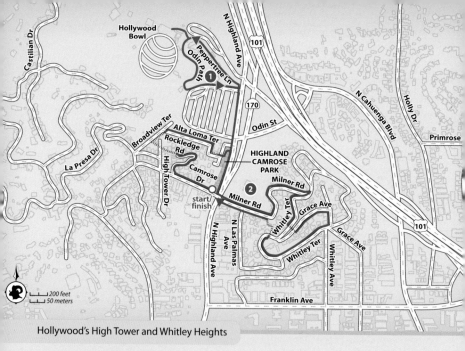

Hollywood's High Tower and Whitley Heights

Points of Interest

1 Hollywood Bowl 2301 N. Highland Ave., Los Angeles, CA 90068; 323-850-2058, hollywoodbowl.com

2 Hollywood Heritage Museum 2100 N. Highland Ave., Hollywood, CA 90068; 323-874-4005, hollywoodheritage.org

The temple at the Vedanta Society of Southern California

16 Lower Beachwood Canyon

BOUNDARIES: Franklin Ave., Ivar Ave., Gower St., Temple Hill Dr.
DISTANCE: About 2 miles
DIFFICULTY: Moderate (includes stairways)
PARKING: Free street parking is available on Vista del Mar Ave.
NEAREST METRO STATION: Red Line (Hollywood Blvd. and Vine St.)

You can't get much more Hollywood than Beachwood Canyon. Situated in the hills immediately below the legendary sign, this neighborhood is home to rising young stars and
accomplished entertainment-industry professionals as well as aging Hollywood burnouts
and struggling actors. This disparate community is reflected in the buildings that line the
narrow streets: an interesting juxtaposition of beautifully maintained million-plus-dollar
houses and rundown 1960s-era apartment buildings.

A word of caution to dog walkers: The narrow and winding streets of this hillside neighborhood can be fairly busy; vehicles tend to materialize around blind curves with little
advance notice, and sidewalks are scarce. Therefore, it's wise to keep your wits about you
and your furry friend on a short leash.

Walk Description

Begin on Vista del Mar Avenue, north of Franklin Avenue, just before the road curves to the right. Straight ahead you'll see a wide double staircase.

Ascend the stairway, which was once grand and lovely but has become somewhat dilapidated over the years. At the top of the steps, you see a towering white mansion across the street at 6215 Holly Mont Drive. This is the onetime home of Golden Age actress Barbara Stanwyck. Like the stairway you just ascended, it appears to have fallen from its former glory, but it still stands in reasonably good condition. Now known as "Holly Mont Castle," the Spanish Revival estate is rumored to be haunted.

Stairway at Vista del Mar Avenue

Turn right on Holly Mont and follow it a short distance to Vista del Mar.

Turn left on Vista del Mar. At 2117–2121 is an apartment building with a sign displaying a pyramid symbol and the words KROTONA OF OLD HOLLYWOOD. This structure is one of several buildings in this area left over from the days of the Krotona Colony, part of the early-20th-century Theosophical movement that melded elements of spiritualism, Eastern religion, Masonic lore, and scientific speculation. Across the street is another remnant of the Krotona Colony—the former Krotona Inn, which incorporates elements of Moorish design, particularly in the domed house that is set back from the street.

Turn right on Primrose Avenue, and continue one short block to Gower Street.

Turn left on Gower. At 2122 Gower, look for a small, modern house that incorporates rounded and rectangular shapes to unique effect. The front gate and garage door are painted in primary colors, completing the home's pleasingly kindergarten-like appearance.

Upon reaching Scenic Avenue, notice the impressive French Normandy–style apartment complex on the northeast corner. Turn left on Scenic, where the homes are consistently well maintained and attractive, encompassing a variety of architectural styles. A Tudor Revival house, partially obscured by bamboo, sits at 6111 Scenic; across the street is an English cottage with an undulating thatched roof.

Cross Vista del Mar Avenue, and continue uphill, as the road curves left. An attractive Spanish Colonial Revival home in dark-stained wood and pale stucco with nicely integrated tile work catches the eye at 6220.

Turn right on Primrose Avenue, and head slightly uphill. Pass Argyle Avenue and follow Primrose downhill. You may catch sight of the hilltop cross known as the Hollywood Pilgrimage Memorial Monument in the middle distance ahead.

Turn left on Alcyona Drive—a NOT A THROUGH STREET sign makes it easy to spot.

When you reach the end of the cul-de-sac, keep an eye out for the hidden stairway and then descend the shady steps to Vine Way.

Continue straight on Vine Way to Vine Street.

Turn left on Vine Street, and follow it one block to Ivar Avenue.

Turn right on Ivar. As Ivar curves around to the left, the street narrows and the sound of rushing traffic indicates that you're approaching US 101. At 2062 Ivar, notice the towering home built in the style of a medieval castle, often referred to as Castle Ivar.

Continue past the intersection with Longview Avenue and then turn left on Vedanta Terrace, immediately before the freeway overpass.

Nearby and Notable: Franklin Village

A few blocks east of the starting point of this walk, Franklin Village—on Franklin Avenue between Tamarind and Bronson Avenues (across the street from the Scientology Celebrity Centre)—is a collection of unique, independently owned businesses that cater to the residents of Beachwood Canyon. The popular strip is home to some decent eateries, such as **Birds** and **La Poubelle**, as well as the **Bourgeois Pig** coffeehouse, **Counterpoint Records & Books**, and the **Upright Citizens Brigade Theatre**—a great spot to discover up-and-coming improv comedians. (See page 79 for street addresses and contact info.)

When you reach the intersection with Vedanta Place, turn right to take a quick detour to the ❶ **Vedanta Society of Southern California** complex, at 1946 Vedanta Place, which features a bookstore and a white temple that looks like a mini Taj Mahal. The Vedanta Society is an ancient religious philosophy based on the sacred scriptures of India known as the Vedas. The temple is open to the public daily for meditation, classes, lectures, and seminars. After checking out the temple, return to Vedanta Terrace and turn right.

Turn left on Vine Street and look over your shoulder to the south to see the top of the distinctive Capitol Records building on the other side of the freeway. At 2030 Vine is a lovely Spanish Mission–style home with a little bell set into the arch over the front gate. You can hear a fountain trickling inside the hidden courtyard.

Turn right on Ivarene Avenue.

Turn right on Alcyona Drive. A charming fairy-tale home sits at 2156 Alcyona.

Turn left on Primrose Avenue, heading back up the hill you descended earlier.

Turn left on Argyle Avenue at the top of the hill.

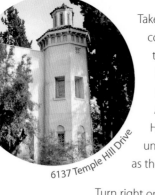

6137 Temple Hill Drive

Take the first right onto Temple Hill Drive. On the northeast corner at 2172 Argyle, notice the huge home that brings to mind a vacation lodge in the mountains. Temple Hill Drive has a mildly rustic air—it's so high in the hills that the freeway and streets of Hollywood seem far away. A modern Moorish mansion stands out at 6191 Temple Hill. The sense of removal from the city lasts until an unexpected view of downtown Los Angeles materializes as the road turns southeast.

Turn right on Vista del Mar Avenue, where Temple Hill ends. Continue downhill along the curving street, and take note of the various architectural styles: Spanish, English, Tudor, Moorish, modern. Such variety lends a whimsical feel to this well-known haven for creative types.

At the intersection with Vista del Mar Place, turn left to stay on Vista del Mar Avenue. Cross Scenic Avenue and Primrose Avenue, retracing your steps down to Holly Mont Drive. Instead of turning on Holly Mont to descend the stairway from the beginning of the walk, remain on Vista del Mar as it curves to the right, taking you back to the beginning of your journey.

If you're feeling peckish, you can continue one block south to the ❷ 101 Coffee Shop, a retro-themed landmark diner on the ground floor of the Best Western hotel at the corner of Vista del Mar and Franklin Avenues.

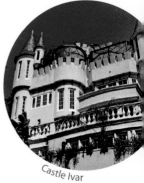

Castle Ivar

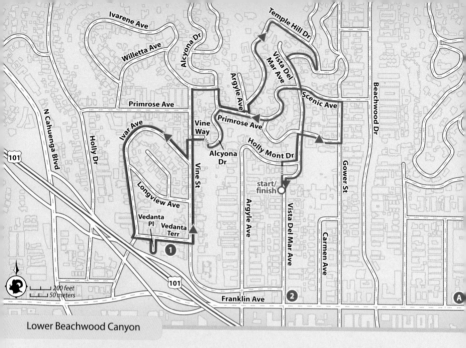

Lower Beachwood Canyon

Points of Interest

1 Vedanta Society of Southern California 1946 Vedanta Place, Hollywood, CA 90068; 323-465-7114, vedanta.org

2 101 Coffee Shop 6145 Franklin Ave., Los Angeles, CA 90028; 323-467-1175, 101coffeeshop.com

A *Franklin Village (see "Nearby and Notable," page 77):*

Bourgeois Pig 5931 Franklin Ave., Los Angeles, CA 90028; 323-464-6008

Birds 5925 Franklin Ave., Los Angeles, CA 90028; 323-465-0175, birdshollywood.com

Upright Citizens Brigade Theatre 5919 Franklin Ave., Los Angeles, CA 90028; 323-908-8702, ucbtheatre.com

Counterpoint Records & Books 5911 Franklin Ave., Los Angeles, CA 90028; 323-957-7965, counterpointla.com

La Poubelle 5907 Franklin Ave., Los Angeles, CA 90028; 323-465-0807, lapoubellebistro.com

The gateway to Hollywoodland

17 Upper Beachwood Canyon and Hollywoodland

BOUNDARIES: Franklin Ave., US 101, Griffith Park
DISTANCE: About 2 miles
DIFFICULTY: Strenuous (includes stairways)
PARKING: Free parking is available on Beachwood Dr.

Beachwood Canyon works hard to maintain its rural, small-town vibe, even though it looks out over frenetic Hollywood. The neighborhood's origins reflect this conceit; in 1923, real estate magnate S. H. Woodruff developed the rustic hills north of Hollywood, which he topped off with an ostentatious four-story sign dubbing it HOLLYWOODLAND. The last four letters have since been removed, and the remainder of the sign—now one of the most recognizable Southern California landmarks in the world—has been treated to the occasional face-lift over the past 80 years (this is Hollywood, after all).

At the time of development, Woodruff hired European stonemasons to construct roadside walls and six long stairways out of wrought iron and stone to connect the residential streets of Hollywoodland. This walk seeks out and conquers every one of these steep flights, so be sure to bring plenty of water and wear comfy shoes.

Walk Description

Begin on Beachwood Drive, just south of Belden Drive, and head north into the canyon. The original stone gates of Hollywoodland sit on either side of the road, and a street sign welcomes residents home while imploring them to SLOW DOWN AND RELAX. To the right, at 2700 Westshire Drive, is the original Hansel and Gretel–style cottage that still houses the Hollywoodland Realty Company.

Turn left on Belden Drive and walk past the neighborhood hub, where locals grab breakfast at ❶ **Beachwood Cafe,** do light grocery shopping at the ❷ **Beachwood Market,** and stay current on the community happenings posted on the bulletin board.

Turn right on Woodshire Drive, a narrow, winding street with a pleasing rustic feel that you follow past flawless Spanish homes, many with stained-glass details in the windows. An imposing Norman castle–style home at 2755 Woodshire catches the eye. Next door is an ivy-covered English cottage with a coat of arms painted over the front door. While the predominant architectural style in the canyon is Mediterranean, the Anglo influence is also apparent.

Just before 2795 Woodshire, look for the first of the somewhat hidden Hollywoodland stairways on your left, and ascend it.

Emerge back on Belden Drive, and turn left.

Citrus trees add a splash of color.

When you reach the fork in the road, bear right to continue uphill on Flagmoor Place. About halfway up the short street, a clearing on the left treats you to a great view of downtown's high-rises to the southeast.

As you approach the intersection of Flagmoor Place and Durand Drive, you can catch an unobstructed view of Griffith Observatory directly to the east. Bear left slightly to head uphill on Durand. You'll notice a great stone wall on your right. Follow this to the front of the magnificent home at 2869 Durand, which was built in the style of a Norman castle.

Cross in front of the entrance to 2869 Durand, and take a few
steps down the dirt trail that lies next to a small parking area
to reach a trailhead. The Lake Hollywood Reservoir sparkles
below and can be reached by following the trail about
0.5 mile downhill.

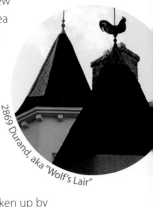

2869 Durand, aka "Wolf's Lair"

Retrace your steps from the trail back to Durand Drive,
and turn left on Durand—back the way you came. Now
heading north, you pass the intersection with Flagmoor
Place, taking care to stay on Durand. The HOLLYWOOD sign
looms large directly ahead.

Just past 2954 Durand is the second stairway, which is broken up by
pathways and landings. Follow the steps all the way down to the street below. Use
caution, as some of the stairs have eroded over time. At the bottom of the steps,
cross Rodgerton Drive to continue straight on Belden Drive.

Follow Belden as it curves east, and look for the next stairway, just past
2950 Belden. This straight, narrow flight, divided by what used to be small ponds
but are now sand-filled planters, is perhaps the most recognizable stairway in
Beachwood Canyon. Descend the steps and then turn left on Woodshire Drive at
the bottom. A bronze Los Angeles Cultural Heritage Commission sign at the
base declares Hollywoodland's granite retaining walls and interconnecting stairways a Historic-Cultural Monument.

Cross Beachwood Drive and turn right on the other side of the street. Between
2800 and 2810 Beachwood is another very long stairway. Take a deep breath
and ascend the 144 steps to Westshire Drive. Again, watch out for cracks and holes
in the 80-year-old concrete.

Turn left at the top of the stairs, and follow Westshire Drive downhill to where
it merges with Beachwood Drive. Notice that some of the homes on the right
appear to have maintained the original stone retaining walls.

Continue north on Beachwood, past vibrantly painted Spanish homes, charming
traditional wood-and-brick houses, and faux castles; the residence at 2925 even

features a large mural of a medieval knight on the wall facing the street. As you approach the intersection with Belden Drive, notice the particularly adorable English cottage at 2958, complete with low stone walls and a thatched-style roof.

Pass Belden Drive and continue on Beachwood, keeping an eye out for the next staircase, which lies on your right between 3020 and 3030 Beachwood. Begin your ascent of the longest stairway of this walk—176 steps—pausing as needed to catch your breath. The houses on either side have particularly large lots, lending a nice rustic feel to this portion of the walk.

At the top of the stairs, turn right on Hollyridge Drive for the longest stairway-free stretch of this route. Thankfully, the road slopes gently downhill here, providing some relief after the no-nonsense sets of stairs you have climbed. Many of the homes on the hill to your left are concealed behind dense foliage, but you can catch glimpses of several interesting styles, including another stone castle and a few imposing contemporary residences. Continue straight on Hollyridge past the intersection with Lechner Place.

At the intersection with Pelham Place, just past 2831 Hollyridge and across the street from another castlelike facade, turn right to descend the final stairway of your journey.

At the bottom of the steps, turn left to follow Westshire Drive about a block back to Beachwood Drive.

Turn left to return to your starting point next to the stone gates marking the entrance to Hollywoodland.

Atop Mount Lee since 1923

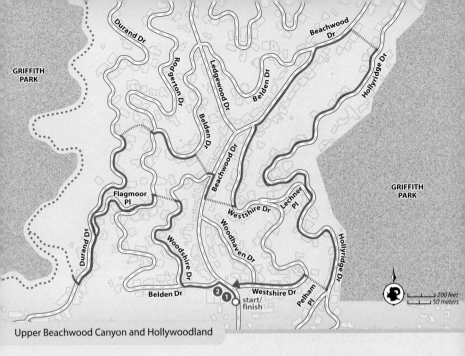

Upper Beachwood Canyon and Hollywoodland

Points of Interest

1 **Beachwood Cafe** 2695 N. Beachwood Drive, Los Angeles, CA 90068; 323-871-1717, beachwoodcafe.com

2 **Beachwood Market** 2701 Belden Drive, Los Angeles, CA 90068; 323-464-7154

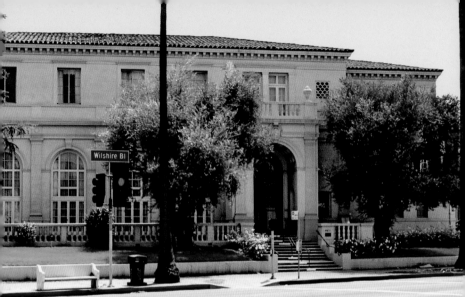

The Ebell of Los Angeles, a women's club, also serves as a wedding and event venue.

18 Larchmont Village and Windsor Square

BOUNDARIES: Beverly Blvd., Rossmore Ave., Wilshire Blvd., Windsor Blvd.
DISTANCE: About 2 miles
DIFFICULTY: Easy
PARKING: Free street parking is available on Larchmont Blvd., south of First St.;
metered parking is available on Larchmont north of First St.

The Hancock Park/Windsor Square area lies just south of Hollywood and is considered one of the nicest areas in central Los Angeles. It encompasses posh Wilshire Country Club, as well as Larchmont Village, a collection of small, independently owned shops and restaurants (as well as a few commercial chain establishments) that is constantly teeming with residents and their canine companions. This route begins in the village and heads south to explore the homes of Windsor Square, a wealthy neighborhood that the city of Los Angeles declared a Historic Preservation Overlay Zone (HPOZ) in 2005. There was some dispute among the residents of Windsor Square over this declaration. The HPOZ designation can be a blessing in that it protects the houses and ensures that the architectural integrity and cohesiveness of all the buildings in the area are carefully upheld, but it can also be limiting to residents who wish to make their own unique mark on their property.

Walk Description

Begin at the corner of Beverly and Larchmont Boulevards, in the middle of Larchmont Village, which stretches for several blocks between Melrose Avenue and Third Street. Head south on Larchmont. The village is home to more restaurants than you can shake a fork at, ranging from Italian to Greek to Thai to Caribbean. Sartorial enthusiasts will be delighted to find a collection of fine boutiques, although the names on some of the storefronts seem to change regularly. It's worth your time either before or after this walk to explore Larchmont Village and grab a bite to eat—if you can decide where to dine. A few long-standing and dependably good eateries include ❶ **Prado Restaurant,** ❷ **Village Pizzeria,** and ❸ **Le Petit Greek.** A more recent arrival is the much-celebrated ❹ **Salt & Straw,** a Portland-import ice-cream shop specializing in unusual and mouthwatering flavor combinations. The popular ❺ **Larchmont Farmers Market** sets up on Sunday mornings in a parking lot on the west side of the street.

Larchmont Boulevard becomes a residential street south of First Street, populated with mostly Spanish and Norman one- and two-story homes. The median is planted with jacaranda, lily of the Nile, and bird-of-paradise. As you near Third Street, look for the stone column erected by the Windsor Square Association at the south end of the Larchmont median.

Cross Third Street and turn left, walking less than a block to Plymouth Boulevard.

Turn right on Plymouth, a quiet street lined with royal palms. The houses here are more appropriately described as mansions, with expansive green lawns and self-conscious ornamentation, such as diamond-paned windows and gingerbread trim. The primary architectural styles are those that work well on a grand scale, such as American Colonial Revival, Spanish Colonial Revival, Craftsman, and Tudor Revival.

Turn right on Wilshire Boulevard. The commanding structure of the Scottish Rite Masonic Temple sits on the northwest corner of Plymouth and Wilshire. On the south side of Wilshire is the Wilshire United Methodist Church, a beautiful building that combines elements of Romanesque and Gothic design and has been declared a Historic-Cultural Monument by the city of Los Angeles. The Italian

Renaissance–style headquarters for ❻ **The Ebell of Los Angeles,** just west of the church, at the corner of Lucerne Boulevard, encompasses the Wilshire Ebell Theatre and Clubhouse. Founded in 1894, The Ebell is one of the nation's oldest and largest women's clubs. The theater and clubhouse were built in 1927.

Turn right on Lucerne Boulevard. At 637 Lucerne, notice a Victorian mansion. Across the street, at 630, is an elaborate Craftsman shingled in green wood. Apart from these two remarkable structures, most of the homes along Lucerne echo the architectural styles of Plymouth.

Turn right on Fourth Street.

Turn left on Windsor Boulevard. A classic white American Colonial Revival home sits on the northeast corner at 354 Windsor.

Carefully cross Third Street; the street is fairly busy, and there's no crosswalk at Windsor. At 270 S. Windsor, a cheerful orange Spanish home with blue-and-yellow-striped awnings catches the eye. As you continue along Windsor, you'll see that many of the gardens are planted with white roses and purple lily of the Nile; the landscaping along this street is impressively congruous. Even in the dry heat of summer, Windsor Boulevard smells verdant, thanks to the blooming magnolia trees and amply watered lawns, although the prolonged SoCal drought is gradually prompting some residents to switch over to low-water landscaping.

Turn left on First Street. The Spanish-style home on the northwest corner looks like a tropical resort, gorgeously landscaped with palms and exotic flowering plants. As you cross Plymouth Boulevard for the last time, look north to catch a glimpse of the water tower at Paramount Studios.

When you come to the intersection of Beachwood Drive, veer left to remain on First Street and take the next right (you'll see Gower Street on the right). Continue on First to the intersection of Larchmont Boulevard.

Turn right on Larchmont and head one block back to Beverly Boulevard, where you started in Larchmont Village.

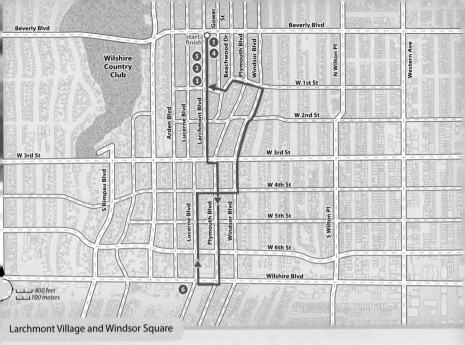

Larchmont Village and Windsor Square

Points of Interest

1 **Prado Restaurant** 244 N. Larchmont Blvd., Los Angeles, CA 90004; 323-467-3871, pradola.com

2 **Village Pizzeria** 131 N. Larchmont Blvd., Los Angeles, CA 90004; 323-465-5566, villagepizzeria.net

3 **Le Petit Greek** 127 N. Larchmont Blvd., Los Angeles, CA 90004; 323-464-5160, lepetitgreek.com

4 **Salt & Straw** 240 N. Larchmont Blvd., Los Angeles, CA 90004; 323-466-0485, saltandstraw.com

5 **Larchmont Farmers Market** 209 N. Larchmont Blvd., Los Angeles, CA 90004; Sundays 10 a.m.–2 p.m.

6 **The Ebell of Los Angeles** 743 S. Lucerne Blvd., Los Angeles, CA 90005; 323-931-1277, ebellla.org

The Wiltern Theatre is an Art Deco masterpiece.

19 Koreatown and Wilshire Center

BOUNDARIES: Western Ave., Wilshire Blvd., Catalina St., Seventh St.
DISTANCE: About 1.5 miles
DIFFICULTY: Easy
PARKING: Metered street parking is available on Western Ave.
NEAREST METRO STATION: Wilshire Blvd. and Western Ave., or Wilshire Blvd. and
   Normandie Ave. (Purple Line)

The area known as Koreatown or Wilshire Center truly has it all: historic buildings, a wealth of dining and shopping options, churches, a giant spa and sports club, and a sizzling night scene. The neighborhood even features two convenient Metro subway stations, making it easy to get here and spend day and night without worrying about parking fees (or designating a driver, should that become an issue). While the area is home to a mostly Korean-American population and many of the businesses cater primarily to Korean-speaking clientele, it has plenty to offer anyone else looking for an adventure, a dose of Los Angeles history, or a taste of authentic Korean culture.

Walk Description

Begin at the corner of Wilshire Boulevard (south side of the street) and Western Avenue, in front of the ❶ **Wiltern Theatre** (the Wilshire/Western Metro station is located directly across the street). This green terra-cotta Art Deco structure opened as an office building and movie theater in 1931 and has since been renovated and declared a Los Angeles Historic-Cultural Monument. Today the venue hosts a variety of performances, from comedy acts to garage bands. Take a minute to check out the underside of the flashy metal and neon marquee, which is decorated with an ornate sunburst design in plaster, and the beautiful carved mahogany doors of the theater lobby.

Just past the imposing Wilshire Park Place office building, ❷ **Aroma Spa and Sports** occupies the southeast corner of the intersection with Serrano Avenue; its *Blade Runner*–esque electronic billboard lures passersby to try out the exclusive club's saunas, spa treatments, four-story driving range, and other sports facilities.

Cross to the north side of Wilshire Boulevard at Serrano Avenue, and continue east. You'll pass the ❸ **Wilshire Boulevard Temple** on the northeast corner of Wilshire and Hobart. Built in 1929, this striking, Byzantine-influenced structure is listed on the National Register of Historic Places. The building's exterior is dominated by a massive dome 100 feet in diameter. If the synagogue is open to the public at the time of your visit, take time to explore the interior, which is decorated in gold and black Italian marble and features murals depicting the biblical story of creation.

After crossing Harvard Boulevard, you'll come upon St. Basil Roman Catholic Church (established in 1969), an imposing building whose vertical concrete panels are interspersed with jagged columns of colorful stained glass, giving it the slightly discordant feel of a Picasso painting.

At ❹ **BCD Tofu House,** on the northeast corner of Wilshire and Kingsley Drive, you can get a table full of *banchan* (assorted Korean salads and pickles) to go with your delicious bubbling bowl of *soon* (a flavorful stew served with tofu and your choice of meat, fish, or vegetables), all for under $10. It's even open 24 hours.

The chic **⑤ Line Hotel** is found at the northwest corner of Wilshire and Normandie Avenue. Besides its hip rooms for guests, the place offers bars, a Poketo boutique, and one heck of a setting for public dining at Commissary, inside a greenhouse set next to the pool.

At the northeast corner of Wilshire and Normandie Avenue is the Oasis Church, an ornate Romanesque structure built in 1927. Cross Normandie; then cross to the south side of Wilshire, and continue east. From this side of the street, you have a better view of the white Art Deco building just east of Wilshire Christian Church, which houses the Consulate General of the Republic of Indonesia. On your right, pass a variety of small, inexpensive eateries, including a popular New York City import, The Halal Guys. This area is bustling with office workers on weekdays.

After crossing Mariposa Avenue, note Wilshire Center's tallest structure, the modernist Equitable Life Building, which towers over the opposite side of the boulevard.

The northeast corner of Wilshire and Alexandria Avenue is the former site of the first of the legendary hat-shaped Brown Derby restaurants—where the Cobb salad is thought to have originated—but the site is now occupied by a cheesy-looking strip mall (named Brown Derby Plaza in honor of the former Hollywood Golden Age hot spot). Just east of the plaza are the 1920s-era Gaylord Apartments, named for Henry Gaylord Wilshire, the millionaire who developed what is now called MacArthur Park. According to popular lore, Wilshire Boulevard was so named because Wilshire would only allow a boulevard to bisect his property if it bore his name. Inside the Gaylord building is the **⑥ HMS Bounty,** one of the city's most noted dive bars.

Another view of the Wiltern

On the south side of the street is the former site of the Ambassador Hotel, the legendary playground for Hollywood's rich and famous and the infamous site of Robert F. Kennedy's assassination. The hotel and its Cocoanut Grove nightclub opened in 1921 and enjoyed decades of fame as a beautiful people's mecca before Sirhan Sirhan killed Kennedy there on

June 5, 1968. The hotel was demolished in 2006, and the property now belongs to the Los Angeles Unified School District. A sign on the median declares this stretch of Wilshire the Robert F. Kennedy Memorial Parkway.

Retrace your steps to Normandie Avenue and turn left on Normandie/Irolo Street. Another historic apartment building, the Piccadilly, is located at 682 S. Irolo St.

Turn right on Seventh Street, a residential street occupied for the most part by apartment buildings, many of them newer midrises that were built to take advantage of the nearby subway stations. One notable exception is the cute apartment building at 3530 W. Seventh St.—its rounded corners and retro '50s-style architecture bring to mind the fenders of a classic automobile.

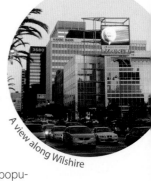

Turn right on Serrano Avenue. You'll notice the netted driving range of Aroma Spa and Sports on your right. The Koreatown branch of the Los Angeles Public Library is on your left.

Cross Wilshire Boulevard and turn left. The curved twin towers of the Wilshire Colonnade office complex on your right are built around a gorgeous circular fountain court-yard—a nice place to enjoy a sandwich or coffee from the popular South Korea–based Tom N Toms that you'll pass in the next block.

A view along Wilshire

Continue two blocks to your starting point at the corner of Wilshire and Western.

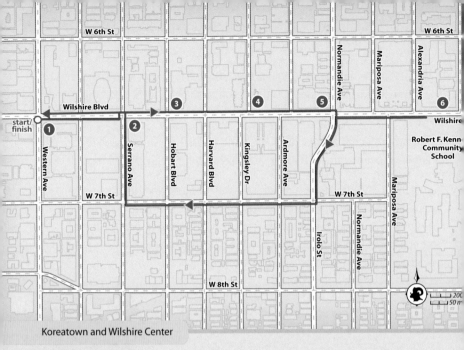

Points of Interest

1. **Wiltern Theatre** 3790 Wilshire Blvd., Los Angeles, CA 90010; 213-380-5005, wiltern.com

2. **Aroma Spa and Sports** 3680 Wilshire Blvd., Los Angeles, CA 90010; 213-387-0212, aromaresort.com

3. **Wilshire Boulevard Temple** 3663 Wilshire Blvd., Los Angeles, CA 90010; 213-388-2401, wbtla.org

4. **BCD Tofu House** 3575 Wilshire Blvd., Los Angeles, CA 90010; 213-382-6677, bcdtofu.com

5. **The Line Hotel** 3515 Wilshire Blvd., Los Angeles, CA 90010; 213-381-7411, thelinehotel.com

6. **HMS Bounty** 3357 Wilshire Blvd., Los Angeles, CA 90010; 213-385-7275

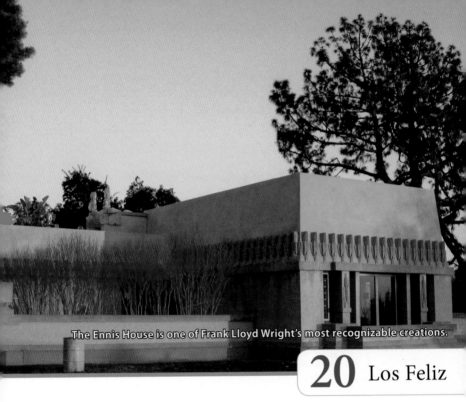

The Ennis House is one of Frank Lloyd Wright's most recognizable creations.

20 Los Feliz

BOUNDARIES: Edgemont St., Glendower Ave., Hillhurst Ave., Sunset Blvd.
DISTANCE: About 1.5–3.5 miles (depending on route chosen)
DIFFICULTY: Strenuous (includes stairways)
PARKING: Free street parking is available on Catalina St.
NEAREST METRO STATION: Vermont Ave. and Sunset Blvd. (Red Line).
  Note: Change the starting point of the walk to Barnsdall Art Park if you take the Metro.

Los Feliz, a charming, vibrant neighborhood just northeast of Hollywood, has fast become an exclusive address, particularly in the hills, and the rest of the region is quickly gentrifying as homebuyers come to appreciate the area's proximity to both the wilderness of Griffith Park and the action of Hollywood and Silver Lake. Fans of Doug Liman's 1996 movie, *Swingers*, will recognize a couple of the nightspots featured prominently in the film: The Dresden Restaurant and the former Derby swing club, along Los Feliz's main drags.

This neighborhood is also notable for its architecture, in particular Frank Lloyd Wright's Ennis House, which is tucked high in the hills, and the architect's Hollyhock House, which sits just over a mile south in the flatlands. This route takes you into Los Feliz's affluent, hilly residential area before making an optional detour south through Los Feliz Village to Barnsdall Art Park, home of the Hollyhock House.

Walk Description

Begin at the corner of Los Feliz Boulevard and Catalina Street, and head north on Catalina. The quiet, magnolia-lined street features attractive, expensive-looking homes. Look up to your left to see the Griffith Observatory, which appears surprisingly close in the hills above.

Turn right on Cromwell Avenue and look for the historic Los Feliz Heights Steps on your left, across the street from 2251 Berendo St.

Ascend the 180 steps, which are shaded in places by overhanging oleander and bougainvillea bushes. About two-thirds of the way up, you'll come to a landing with thoughtfully built-in benches.

At the top of the stairs, turn right on Bonvue Avenue and follow the narrow road as it winds higher into the hills. Keep an eye out for cars around the sharp bend. This street has a very Mediterranean feel, with magnificent two- and three-story Spanish homes built into the hill on the left.

Eventually, you come to a split in the road. Continue straight on what is now Glendower Avenue and prepare for numerous architectural feats. At 2567, you pass the Skolnik House, one of architect Rudolph Schindler's last designs, but you can't see much of the building apart from the shimmering green outer wall. Across the street at 2574, find the Witches Whimsy, a relic from the 1920s, when the short-lived Storybook style became popular in Los Angeles. A few doors down, at 2587, is another eye-catching house; composed of metal and gray concrete, the industrial-looking structure towers over the road, supported by sturdy-looking cement columns. Finally, at 2607 Glendower, you reach the start of Frank Lloyd Wright's imposing and innovative ❶ **Ennis House**, one of the architect's four textile-block designs in the LA area. This massive structure, built in 1924, overlooks the

Designer Name: Frank Lloyd Wright

Born in 1867, Frank Lloyd Wright is probably America's best-known architect, renowned for masterpieces as diverse as the Guggenheim Museum in New York City and the Fallingwater residence in western Pennsylvania. Inspired by the wide-open prairies of his birthplace in Wisconsin, Wright introduced the ideas of open floor plans and organic design in residential architecture.

In the early 1920s, Wright pioneered his concrete textile block style in Southern California. This innovative technique involved using premanufactured engraved concrete blocks that were inset with glass to allow light to filter indoors. One advantage of this system was affordability, as concrete blocks made a cheap, modular building material. There are four examples of Wright's textile-block architecture in the Los Angeles area: the Ennis House in Los Feliz, the Millard House in Pasadena, and the Samuel Freeman and John Storer Houses in the Hollywood Hills.

Los Angeles basin below and is constructed of cinder blocks carved with Mayan designs, giving it the look of an ancient fortress.

Follow Glendower as it curves around the Ennis House, eventually lending a view of the north-facing facade of the home. The building is perhaps most recognizable as the home of Harrison Ford's character in *Blade Runner*, although it's been featured in many other films. Continue west on Glendower. With their eclectic mix of architectural styles, the homes on this high, sunny street boast spectacular views of the city below.

Just before you reach 2763 Glendower, you'll see a signpost reading PUBLIC WALK. Descend these stairs down to Bryn Mawr Road, pausing to admire the stunning vista of the hills to the northeast and of the Ennis House to your left.

Cross the cul-de-sac and continue down the next set of steps to Bonvue Avenue. This stairway is enhanced by a colorful tiled mural that was funded by the Los Feliz Improvement Association.

At the bottom of the steps, cross the street to go straight on Glendower Avenue. Follow the winding road as it gently leads downhill past more beautiful homes.

Continue to follow the road as it curves sharply to the right, and bypass Glendower Place, which branches off to the left.

Glendower merges with Vermont Avenue, which leads up to the Greek Theatre, a moderate-sized outdoor concert venue. Continue south on Vermont.

At this point, you can either turn right on Los Feliz Boulevard and head a few blocks west to your starting point at Catalina Street, or you can continue through Los Feliz Village to the Barnsdall Art Park, home of Frank Lloyd Wright's Hollyhock House. This optional route is detailed next.

Addendum

Cross Los Feliz Boulevard and continue south on Vermont Avenue into Los Feliz Village. The first few blocks along Vermont consist mostly of apartment buildings and a few houses of worship. But after you cross Franklin Avenue, it becomes more interesting. The thriving collection of shops and restaurants along the next few blocks includes House of Pies, a middling family restaurant with a huge selection of doughy desserts; ❷ **Palermo Ristorante Italiano,** where vino flows freely in the waiting lounge on busy nights; ❸ **Fred 62,** a retro diner for hipsters; the Los Feliz 3 Cinemas; independent ❹ **Skylight Books;** Squaresville vintage clothing store; the legendary ❺ **Dresden Restaurant;** the classy Vermont Restaurant and Bar; and several more casual and upscale eateries, chic clothing shops, and home-decor boutiques. It's amazing how many commercial points of interest are crammed into this short stretch.

Turn right on Prospect Avenue, which merges with Hollywood Boulevard, to enter the Little Armenia neighborhood.

Cross the street at New Hampshire Avenue, and enter ❻ **Barnsdall Art Park,** on the south side of Hollywood Boulevard. This innovative community arts center atop Olive Hill is virtually hidden from the streets below. In addition to the

Los Angeles Municipal Arts Gallery and Junior Arts Center, the park is home to another Frank Lloyd Wright masterpiece, the Hollyhock House.

Ascend the stairs into the park, turn right at the second road, and then ascend the next set of steps on your left to a beautiful, grassy park dotted with pine trees.

If you'd like to learn more about the art programs at the park, you can do so at the municipal art gallery on the left. Otherwise, continue straight along the path through the park, and then turn right to reach the Hollyhock House. This was Wright's first project in Los Angeles, predating the Ennis House by several years. Wright used this project to create a regionally appropriate architectural style, which he referred to as California Romanza. This style interweaves indoor and outdoor space, making extensive use of rooftop terraces and enclosed gardens. If you wish to go inside the house, which was restored and reopened in 2015, there is a fee.

After exploring the park, begin to retrace your steps to Hollywood Boulevard, but before you get too far, look north to take in your accomplishment so far: you should be able spot the Ennis House, as well as the HOLLYWOOD sign and Griffith Observatory.

Cross the street at New Hampshire Avenue and turn right to retrace your steps along Prospect Avenue.

Cross Vermont Avenue and continue east on Prospect, passing several old wooden houses and a collection of apartment buildings.

Turn left on Hillhurst Avenue. This isn't exactly the most enticing street, but it features numerous restaurants, bars, and coffeehouses that are popular with both locals and out-of-towners. For some of the most popular tacos in town, hop a block south to **7 The Best Fish Taco in Ensenada** at 1650 Hillhurst. At 1760, you pass Home, a—you guessed it—*home*-style outdoor eatery that offers a few healthy twists on your traditional diner menu. At 1831, you encounter Ye Rustic Inn, a dive bar in a strip mall that has proved inexplicably popular with trend-seeking scenesters and neighborhood drunks alike. **8 Alcove Cafe & Bakery** tempts passersby with a welcoming patio and a tantalizing array of baked goodies at 1929, as does Jeni's Splendid Ice Creams (of Columbus, Ohio, fame) at 1954 Hillhurst.

Near Los Feliz Boulevard are more food-and-drink venues: Mexico City, a decent midpriced eatery that serves stiff margaritas, and Messhall Kitchen, a gastropub that unfortunately replaced the Derby, the swing-dancing club immortalized in the film *Swingers,* which provided a humorous glimpse into the nightlife of Hollywood's struggling actors on the brink of the late-'90s swing-dancing craze. For those interested in beauty and wellness, this stretch of Hillhurst also features an intimate neighborhood spa, ❾ **Being in LA,** at 2122 Hillhurst.

Turn left on Los Feliz Boulevard. After you cross Vermont Avenue, the homes on either side of the street become increasingly opulent. Continue for three more short blocks back to your starting point at the corner of Los Feliz and Catalina Street.

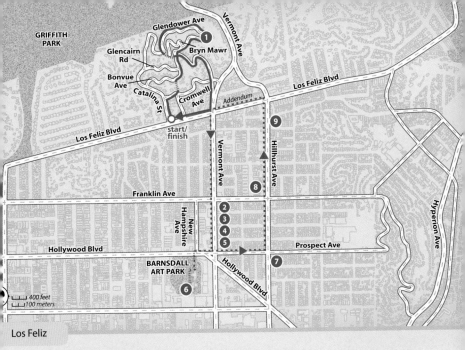

Los Feliz

Points of Interest

1 Ennis House 2607 Glendower Ave., Los Angeles, CA 90027

Addendum:

2 Palermo Ristorante Italiano 1858 N. Vermont Ave., Los Angeles, CA 90027; 323-663-1178, palermorestaurant.net

3 Fred 62 1850 N. Vermont Ave., Los Angeles, CA 90027; 323-667-0062, fred62.com

4 Skylight Books 1818 N. Vermont Ave., Los Angeles, CA 90027; 323-660-1175, skylightbooks.com

5 The Dresden Restaurant 1760 N. Vermont Ave., Hollywood, CA 90027; 323-665-4294, thedresden.com

6 Barnsdall Art Park/Hollyhock House 4800 Hollywood Blvd., Los Angeles, CA 90027; 323-644-6269

7 The Best Fish Taco in Ensenada 1650 N. Hillhurst Ave., Los Angeles, CA 90027; 323-466-5552, bestfishtacoinensenada.com

8 Alcove Cafe & Bakery 1929 Hillhurst Ave., Los Angeles, CA 90027; 323-644-0100

9 Being in LA 2122 Hillhurst Ave., Los Angeles, CA 90027; 323-741-8035, beinginla.com

The Shakespeare Bridge spanning Franklin Avenue

21 Franklin Hills

BOUNDARIES: Franklin Ave., Fountain Ave., Talmadge St., Hyperion Ave.
DISTANCE: About 0.75 mile
DIFFICULTY: Moderate (includes stairways)
PARKING: Free street parking is available on the north side of Franklin Ave., east of the
Shakespeare Bridge.

Nestled between Los Feliz and Silver Lake, Franklin Hills is another of central Los Angeles's
endearing hilly neighborhoods. This residential area was developed in the 1920s as a
quiet community centrally located in the midst of the sprawling metro area, and today it
retains an old-fashioned, neighborly quality that many of LA's newer developments lack.
This impression is reinforced by the two very long concrete stairways that connect the
region's winding streets, giving neighbors relatively easy walking access to one another's
homes while keeping their hearts and lungs in great condition.

Walk Description

Begin just east of the ❶ **Shakespeare Bridge** on Franklin Avenue. Built in 1926, this distinctive white structure bridged the way, so to speak, for the charming neighborhood of Franklin Hills. Walk to the south side of the street, just past the house that sits immediately east of the bridge, and descend a ficus- and bougainvillea-shaded staircase leading down just beyond the sign for St. George Street.

You emerge in the cul-de-sac at the north end of Sanborn Avenue. Continue south on Sanborn; most of the homes on this street are simple and modern in design, and a few are painted in vibrant colors. On your right, pass a community garden with a variety of vegetables that was planted by the people living here. Behind the garden is the campus of ❷ **The International School of Los Angeles,** a city Historic-Cultural Monument because it was designed by notable Southern California architect John Lautner.

Follow the road as it curves left and becomes Melbourne Avenue. Most of the homes here are modest and well maintained and exhibit a variety of architectural styles: traditional, Spanish Colonial Revival, English country cottage. At 3912 Melbourne is a dramatically different style of home—a fairy-tale English cottage with a deeply sloping wood-shingled roof and diamond-pane windows.

Continue straight across Deloz Avenue and look for the sign for the Radio Walk steps just to the right of 1856 Deloz. Ascend the long staircase, which can feel like a secret passage when overgrown with a thick layer of dead leaves. Cross Hollyvista Avenue and continue up the next flight of steps, which is more heavily shaded than the first half of Radio Walk.

Emerge on Franklin Avenue, just north of Radio Street. Turn right to pass Radio Street and continue on Franklin. You can catch occasional glimpses of the Griffith Observatory between the houses on your right.

Turn right just past 3818 Franklin to descend the Prospect Walk stairway, and pause at the top of the steps to admire the view east along Hollywood Boulevard, which stretches out below. Cross Hollyvista Avenue and continue down the next set of steps.

When you reach Deloz Avenue, turn right instead of descending the last flight of Prospect Walk stairs. Deloz is a quiet, sunny street with lots of cute Spanish-style houses, French and English cottages, and many traditional homes. The houses built into the steeply sloping hill on the right appear to be much larger than those on the left side of the street, but appearances can be deceiving with these hillside homes.

Pass Prospect Avenue and continue on Deloz Avenue, passing the Radio Walk steps you ascended earlier. This is a bit of a tricky intersection, as it marks the connection of Deloz, Prospect, and Melbourne, so be sure to continue straight ahead, hugging the right side of the street, rather than wandering off on one of these offshoots.

Deloz Avenue ends when it merges with Hollyvista Avenue. Continue straight on what is now Hollyvista. At 2024, take note of a delightful home with blue awnings, a wood-shingled roof, and a white picket fence—the picture of blissful domesticity. A large, austere, modern home sits in stark contrast at 2100 Hollyvista.

Turn left at the next intersection to head west on Franklin Avenue, and you will shortly return to your starting point just east of the Shakespeare Bridge.

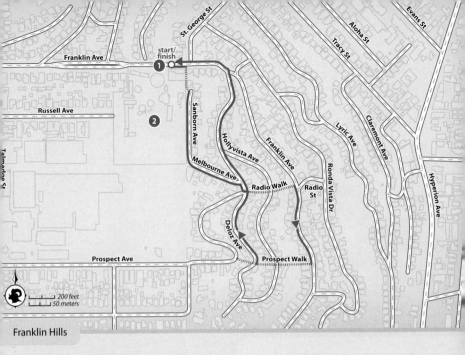

Franklin Hills

Points of Interest

1. **Shakespeare Bridge** Franklin Avenue at Monon Street, Los Angeles, CA 90027

2. **The International School of Los Angeles** 4155 Russell Ave., Los Angeles, CA 90027; 323-665-4526, internationalschool.la

The Los Feliz Cafe feeds hungry golfers at the municipal course.

22 Atwater Village

BOUNDARIES: Los Feliz Blvd., I-5, Glendale Blvd., San Fernando Rd.
DISTANCE: About 2 miles
DIFFICULTY: Easy
PARKING: Free street parking is available on Glenfeliz Blvd.

Sandwiched between Los Feliz and the suburb of Glendale, Atwater Village offers charming residential neighborhoods as well as a burgeoning dining and shopping scene. The neighborhood has long been home to low-key watering holes such as the Roost and Bigfoot Lodge, which attract hip crowds from nearby Hollywood, Silver Lake, and Los Feliz. And the opening of an upscale day spa and a handful of trendy shops and restaurants is only adding to the appeal of this formerly under-the-radar 'hood.

Walk Description

Begin at the corner of Glenfeliz Boulevard and Los Feliz Boulevard, and head south on Glenfeliz, passing an elementary school on your left as you head away from busy Los Feliz Boulevard into a relatively quiet residential neighborhood filled with homes topped with Spanish roofs.

After crossing Dover Street, bear left to remain on Glenfeliz. The street is lined with shady sycamore trees and quaint, modest-sized homes in a predominantly Spanish architectural style.

Turn left on Glendale Boulevard. This stretch of the busy thoroughfare is home to a variety of small businesses; the mix includes everything from dentists and insurance offices to upscale home-furnishings and pet boutiques. Thankfully, there are also some good dining options here. ❶ Indochine Vien, at 3110, serves up mouthwatering *pho* and other affordable Vietnamese tasties, while ❷ Tacos Villa Corona, at 3185, is the spot for what very well may be the best potato tacos you've ever tasted (for just a buck). And if you're in the mood for some retro flavor, stop in at ❸ Club Tee Gee, at 3210, a dive bar that's been around since 1946 and has the decor to match (re-created after a fire destroyed the interior in 1993).

Turn left on Brunswick Avenue. Notice the colorful "fantasy bungalows" at 3642 and 3648. These 1920s homes combine Egyptian and Norman architectural styles to unique and whimsical effect and are so named because their style shows the influence of silent-movie sets from that period. At 3742 is another notable home featuring trapezoidal windows. Apart from these standouts, the street features a hodgepodge of residential architecture, consisting mainly of Craftsman and Mediterranean homes.

Turn right on Dover Street and walk two short blocks to Revere Avenue.

Turn left on Revere.

Turn left on Los Feliz Boulevard. Straight ahead is a large shopping complex featuring a Costco, Toys"R"Us, Best Buy, and various chain restaurants. At 2980 is the Tudor-style ❹ Tam O'Shanter Inn (part of the venerable Lawry's restaurant family), which specializes in prime rib. Inside, waitresses dressed in Scottish tartan serve up tasty fare such as Yorkshire pudding, Toad in the Hole, and, of course, prime rib. While the atmosphere is a bit stuffy and the prices steep, dining here is a unique experience, and the food is undeniably delicious. Walt Disney came here often, and if you're lucky, you might get seated at his favorite spot.

Other notable locations on this stretch of Los Feliz Boulevard include neighborhood watering holes The Griffin, The Roost, and The Bigfoot Lodge, at 3000, 3100, and 3172, respectively; ❺ **India Sweets and Spices,** which features a casual cafeteria where you can snack on tasty vegetarian Indian fare or enjoy a complete meal on the cheap, at 3126; and ❻ **Potted,** a fun and eclectic garden-design shop, at 3158. On the north side of the street is the ❼ **Los Feliz Municipal Golf Course,** an affordable nine-hole course tucked into the corner of Griffith Park, at 3207 Los Feliz Blvd. (You may choose to forgo the links and enjoy a greasy bite at an outdoor table at the course's Los Feliz Cafe.)

Return to your starting point at the corner of Glenfeliz Boulevard. To reward yourself for your nearly 2-mile trek, consider dropping in at ❽ **dtox Day Spa,** just past Glenfeliz at 3206 Los Feliz Blvd. This pampering sanctuary, housed in a beautifully converted industrial space, offers Zen-inspired treatments and all the spa amenities you need to unwind completely.

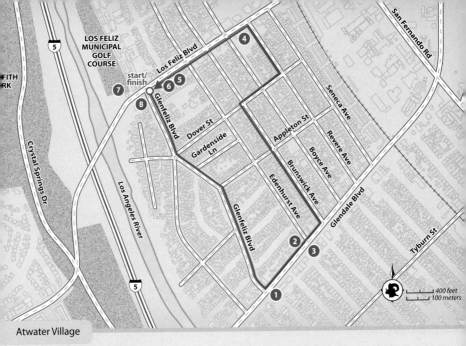

Atwater Village

Points of Interest

1 **Indochine Vien** 3110 Glendale Blvd., Los Angeles, CA 90039; 323-667-9591, indochinevien.com

2 **Tacos Villa Corona** 3185 Glendale Blvd., Los Angeles, CA 90039; 323-661-3458

3 **Club Tee Gee** 3210 Glendale Blvd., Los Angeles, CA 90039; 323-669-9631

4 **Tam O'Shanter Inn** 2980 Los Feliz Blvd., Los Angeles, CA 90039; 323-664-0228, lawrysonline.com/tam-oshanter

5 **India Sweets and Spices** 3126 Los Feliz Blvd., Los Angeles, CA 90039; 323-345-0360, indiasweetsandspices.us

6 **Potted** 3158 Los Feliz Blvd., Los Angeles, CA 90039; 323-665-3801, pottedstore.com

7 **Los Feliz Municipal Golf Course** 3207 Los Feliz Blvd., Los Angeles, CA 90039; 323-663-7758, golf.lacity.org/cdp_los_feliz.htm

8 **dtox Day Spa** 3206 Los Feliz Blvd., Los Angeles, CA 90039; 323-665-3869, dtoxdayspa.com

The Brand Library & Art Center comprises a fanciful hodgepodge of architectural styles.

23 Glendale's Brand Park and Kenneth Village

BOUNDARIES: Brand Park, Grandview Ave., Kenneth Rd., Western Ave.
DISTANCE: About 1.5 miles
DIFFICULTY: Moderate
PARKING: Free parking is available in the Brand Park lot.

Located between Burbank and Pasadena, the city of Glendale bridges the gap between the San Fernando and San Gabriel Valleys. This walk explores two of Glendale's more charming attractions, Brand Park and Kenneth Village. The Brand Library & Art Center, inside Brand Park, was built in 1904 as the home of Leslie Coombs Brand, an early developer in the Glendale area. He named his mansion, perched in the foothills of the Verdugo Mountains, El Miradero, or The Lookout, for its views of the valley below. After exploring the park, head downhill to Kenneth Village, which lends a delightful small-town character to this part of Glendale.

Walk Description

Begin in ❶ **Brand Park,** at the intersection of Mountain Street and Grandview Avenue, where you can spend some time exploring the park and the Brand Library & Art Center. The lovely structure combines elements of Spanish, Moorish, and Indian architecture. Stop in to peruse the library's impressive art and music collections or to admire the latest exhibition in the adjacent gallery. While in the park, you may also want to visit the Whispering Pine Treehouse & Friendship Garden, a lovely little Japanese garden and pond, as well as the Victorian Doctor's House Museum and Gazebo. The Doctor's House was the former residence of three prominent Glendale physicians and has been restored to its late 19th-century appearance.

Exit the park onto Grandview Avenue. A large 1925 Spanish Colonial Revival home named Casa de Carmen catches the eye to your left, at 1770 Mountain St. Head south on Grandview, going slightly downhill away from Brand Park. Notice the homes over the next three blocks: you're in the North Cumberland Heights Historic District, where you can see examples of period revival architectural styles, as well as Minimal Traditional and ranch-style homes. Use the left side of Grandview, as the sidewalk on the right side is intermittent, occasionally pushing pedestrians onto this fairly high-traffic street.

Turn right on Kenneth Road. You're now in the midst of Kenneth Village, Glendale's diminutive, old-fashioned downtown area. This one-block stretch has a pleasing small-town vibe and is home to the ❷ **Village French Bakery,** a yoga studio, a music center, and more.

Turn right on Sonora Avenue. Enjoy the view of the foothills and mountains ahead as you stroll slightly uphill along this residential street. The neighborhood features an eclectic architectural mix—Mediterranean, Norman, Cape Cod, and traditional— and most of the homes have broad green lawns (if it's not a drought year, that is).

Turn left on Bel Aire Drive. This street's residences range in style and size; modest traditional homes stand alongside grand Mediterranean villas. The large wood-shingled house at 1600 Bel Aire, with its steeply pitched roof and stone chimney, catches the eye.

Turn right on El Miradero Avenue. The architecture here is remarkably cohesive, consisting mostly of meticulously maintained Spanish-style homes, many with distinctive flourishes such as colorful tile work and arched picture windows. As you near the end of El Miradero at Mountain Street, you'll see the white Brand Park entrance gate ahead.

Walk through the gate to return to your starting point inside the park.

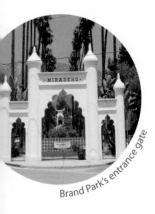

Brand Park's entrance gate

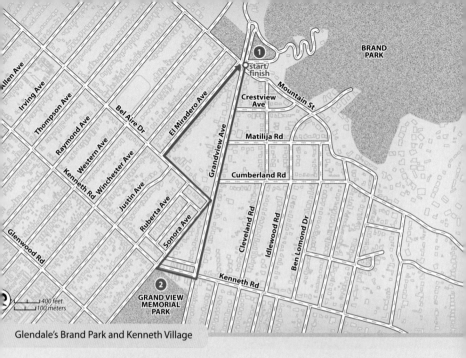

Glendale's Brand Park and Kenneth Village

Points of Interest

1 **Brand Park** 1601 W. Mountain St., Glendale, CA 91201; 818-548-3782, tinyurl.com/brandpark

2 **Village French Bakery** 1414 W. Kenneth Road, Glendale, CA 91201; 818-241-2521

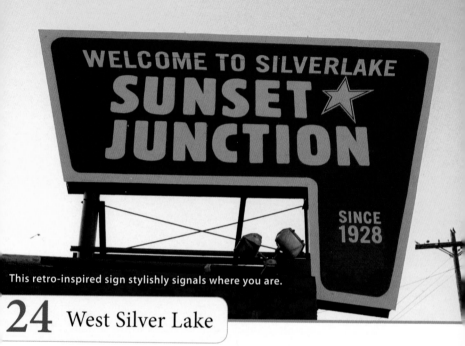

This retro-inspired sign stylishly signals where you are.

24 West Silver Lake

BOUNDARIES: Sunset Blvd., Silver Lake Blvd., Marathon St., Hoover St.
DISTANCE: About 1.75 miles
DIFFICULTY: Moderate (includes stairways)
PARKING: Free street parking is available on Vendome St.

When it comes to hip neighborhoods, Silver Lake is one of the hippest in the country. Often compared with Williamsburg in Brooklyn, New York City, Silver Lake has experienced a cultural/demographic shift over the years, from predominantly Latino to gay to young hipsters and now, with three-room homes renting north of $4,000 a month, increasingly more upper-class and trendy. This walk explores the area's residential streets as well as the main commercial drag along Sunset Boulevard, which offers a cool and eclectic collection of shops, restaurants, and cafés.

Walk Description

Begin at the intersection of Vendome Street and Del Monte Drive, just south of Sunset Boulevard. On the west side of Vendome, across from the intersection of Del Monte, are the famous Music Box Steps, immortalized in Laurel and Hardy's 1932 short film, *The Music Box,* in which the duo attempts to move a piano up the 133 steps and hilarity ensues.

Ascend the staircase to Descanso Drive, climb another short flight of wooden steps to the second level of the split street, and then turn left.

Follow Descanso Drive as it curves to the right. On the northwest corner of Descanso Drive and Micheltorena Street is a cheerful home painted with flowers; the front gate is decorated with a mosaic angel. Continue on Descanso across Micheltorena, and notice how the homes become more attractively maintained as you head farther up the hill.

When you reach the end of Descanso Drive, turn right on Maltman Avenue. Follow the road over the crest of the hill, past a handful of lovely Craftsman homes, and then all the way down to Sunset Boulevard.

Turn left on Sunset. On the opposite side of the street are ❶ **Pine & Crane,** a Taiwanese restaurant just off Sunset on Griffith Park Boulevard; ❷ **El Cóndor,** a hip Mexican restaurant; ❸ **Pazzo Gelato;** and other tempting dining options.

Once you cross Lucile Avenue, the abundance of funky specialty shops is a sure sign of this neighborhood's style of gentrification. Trendy home-furnishings stores line the northeast side of Sunset, while the southwest side features an eclectic array of shops and cafés. Upscale gift shops and baby boutiques sit next door to vintage-clothing stores and the ❹ **Surplus Value Center,** where you can stock up on Dickies gear and fatigues. Cleverly named shops like Den of Antiquity and Bar Keeper (a vintage-barware and liquor store) signal the creativity of Silver Lake's small-business owners.

As you approach Sanborn Avenue, note the SUNSET JUNCTION sign over the sidewalk. ❺ **Intelligentsia,** a gourmet and eco-friendly coffeehouse, holds court at

3922 Sunset. The cluster of shops on the corner, several of which are hidden from the street, includes the Cheese Store of Silver Lake, Cafe Stella, and a flower shop.

Turn around at Sanborn Avenue to retrace your steps back to Maltman Avenue. Cross Maltman and continue along Sunset Boulevard, passing the charming Purgatory Pizza on the corner and ❻ **Millie's,** a no-frills diner frequented by the neighborhood's edgier artists and rockers, located at 3524. The strip mall next door is home to ❼ **Trois Familia,** a breakfast-and-lunch spot that blends French and Mexican.

When you pass Micheltorena Street, look for the short sidewalk that leads to a long stairway on your right; an interesting wooden rotunda sits in the enclosed yard to the left of the sidewalk. Ascend the Micheltorena steps as far as Larissa Drive, and turn left (don't climb the second flight of steps).

Continue along Larissa, keeping right when the road splits, at which point it becomes Descanso Drive.

Follow Descanso Drive uphill, and keep an eye out for the short flight of steps from earlier that cuts across the median on your left.

Descend these steps, and then cross to the other side of the street, back to the Music Box Steps, which you climbed earlier. Head downstairs to return to your starting point on Vendome Street.

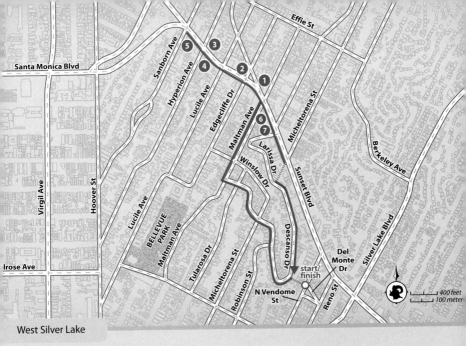

West Silver Lake

Points of Interest

① **Pine & Crane** 1521 Griffith Park Blvd., Los Angeles, CA 90026; 323-668-1128, pineandcrane.com

② **El Cóndor** 3701 W. Sunset Blvd., Los Angeles, CA 90026; 323-660-4500, elcondorla.com

③ **Pazzo Gelato** 3827 W. Sunset Blvd., Los Angeles, CA 90026; 323-662-1710

④ **Surplus Value Center** 3828 W. Sunset Blvd., Los Angeles, CA 90026; 323-662-8132, surplusvaluecenter.net

⑤ **Intelligentsia** 3922 W. Sunset Blvd., Los Angeles, CA 90029; 323-663-6173, intelligentsiacoffee.com

⑥ **Millie's** 3524 W. Sunset Blvd., Los Angeles, CA 90026; 323-664-0404, milliescafela.com

⑦ **Trois Familia** 3510 W. Sunset Blvd., Los Angeles, CA 90026; 323-725-7800, troisfamilia.com

The Richard Neutra–designed O'Hara House

25 East Silver Lake

BOUNDARIES: Silver Lake Blvd., Glendale Blvd., Earl St., Sunset Blvd.
DISTANCE: About 2 miles
DIFFICULTY: Strenuous (includes stairways)
PARKING: Free street parking is available on Silver Lake Blvd.

Silver Lake is a popular destination for LA's gay, artist, and musician communities, as well as for culturally diverse young families who have found that the neighborhood's picturesque hills and lively community spirit make it a desirable alternative to areas such as the beach cities of the Westside or the Hollywood Hills. This route starts in one of the neighborhood's destinations for daytime shopping and nighttime music and then climbs into the hills overlooking the Silver Lake Reservoir, where you'll discover rustic, overgrown walkways and homes that seem so far removed from urban sprawl, you'll hardly believe you're only a few minutes from downtown.

Walk Description

Begin on Silver Lake Boulevard between Berkeley Avenue and Effie Street, and head northeast. For the most part, Silver Lake Boulevard is lined with houses and apartment buildings, but this short stretch features a collection of cute stores and cafés. At ❶ Yolk (1626 Silver Lake Blvd.), you can choose from a selection of hip merchandise such as children's toys, home decorations, architectural books, and yummy-scented candles. Across the street is an elegant interior-design firm, ironically called Rubbish. Neighborhood eateries such as L&E Oyster, Milk, and ❷ LA Mill (an upscale coffeehouse and diner) are good places to consider after this strenuous walk.

❸ The Satellite, Silver Lake's main venue for live music from about-to-break bands, resides at 1717 Silver Lake Blvd. After crossing Van Pelt Place, you'll see where all the dogs you've probably passed came from: the ❹ Silver Lake Recreation Center and off-leash dog park sit at the base of the neighborhood's namesake reservoir, on the north side of the street. At 1886 Silver Lake Blvd. is a fairy-tale Tudor Revival house.

After passing Duane Street, you come to a fork in the road where Rockford Road splits off from Silver Lake Boulevard to the right. Follow Rockford uphill. At 1948 Rockford is a striking modern home with a shallow, peaked roof and jutting eaves over the garage that give the structure a top-heavy look. Next door is a mysterious gated compound with a long stairway that presumably leads up to Apex Avenue, which runs parallel to Rockford. You can catch occasional glimpses down to the sparkling blue reservoir between the houses on your left.

Turn right on Cove Avenue. Look for the wide stairway up ahead, and ascend its shallow steps, stopping to turn and admire the spectacular vista of the reservoir, the hills of Silver Lake, and, in the distance, the HOLLYWOOD sign and the dome of Griffith Observatory. These are the Mattachine Steps, named after the Mattachine Society, founded by Harry Hay, who lived next to the steps. Founded in 1950, the group was one of the first gay-rights organizations in the country.

At the top of the stairs, continue straight on Cove for one more block to Apex Avenue and turn left, following it down the hill toward Glendale Boulevard. Despite the picturesque surroundings, some of the homes in this neighborhood are unkempt, with peeling paint and messy yards.

At the diagonal intersection of Apex Avenue and Glendale Boulevard, *carefully* cross Glendale—there is no crosswalk—and then turn left to head north on Glendale.

Turn right on Loma Vista Place. At 2384, look for the whimsical house with wavy walls and colorful mosaics that bring to mind the architecture of Antoni Gaudí.

Ascend the steps at the end of the cul-de-sac. This combination stairway and walkway may well be the longest one in Los Angeles. Heavily overgrown in places and lined on either side with bungalows and farmhouses, the Loma Vista Place path has a distinctly rural feel. Eventually, the shady staircase widens and starts to head downhill. At this point, you can hear the dull roar of CA 2 just ahead, startling you back into awareness of your urban surroundings.

When you reach the end of the Loma Vista Place stairs, turn left on Allesandro Way, which runs right next to the freeway. Across the freeway, you can see the hills of Elysian Valley.

Turn left on Earl Street and bear right to bypass Earl Court.

When you reach the intersection of Earl Street and Bancroft Avenue, look for a stairway near the street sign. Ascend the Earl Street steps, an extensive, zigzagging stairway.

At the top of the stairs, continue straight on Earl Street, which heads downhill at a sharp angle after it crosses Hidalgo Avenue. As you descend the hill toward Glendale Boulevard, the reservoir comes into view once more.

Once again, *carefully* cross Glendale Boulevard and continue on Earl Street. This stretch of Earl features several architecturally interesting houses. At 2425 is a lovely Spanish home with vibrant blue trim and a mailbox covered in brightly colored tile. At 2434 Earl St., you'll notice a stepped structure covered in weathered wood shingles. This is the Treetops triplex, designed in 1980 by Dion Neutra, son of acclaimed modernist architect Richard Neutra. Next door, at the corner of Earl Street and Neutra Place, shrouded by bamboo and trees, is the headquarters of the Institute for Survival Through Design, run by Dion himself.

Designer Name: Richard Neutra

Born in Vienna in 1892, Richard Neutra came to be one of the leaders of the Southern California modern-architecture movement. After training with Otto Wagner in Austria, Neutra was drawn to the United States by American architectural legend Frank Lloyd Wright and eventually settled in California, where he worked closely with another Viennese-born modernist icon, Rudolph Schindler. Neutra's signature designs consist of a light metal frame with a stucco or wood finish and extensive use of glass, creating an effect that is both light and industrial. His buildings also take advantage of the region's amenable climate by carefully integrating residential landscapes into the structural design.

Neutra found Silver Lake to be LA's most open-minded neighborhood in terms of innovative architecture, so he built his home and studio in the hills overlooking the reservoir, and he also designed several more houses in this neighborhood.

Turn left on Neutra Place. This short cul-de-sac is a showcase of the architecture of Dion's father, Richard. You can see examples of his work at 2218, 2200, and 2210 Neutra Place. The O'Hara House, at 2210, is particularly striking; perched high above the street to afford views of the reservoir through its giant picture windows, the structure is a study of geometric shapes in glass and wood.

Retrace your steps to Earl Street and turn left toward Silver Lake Boulevard.

Turn left on Silver Lake Boulevard. You're now level with the reservoir just across the street, and the Silver Lake Meadow, a passive park space "reserved for quiet enjoyment." This stretch of the boulevard is rather pleasant, shaded with towering pines and eucalyptus trees. As you head south on Silver Lake Boulevard, you pass another string of Richard Neutra–designed homes on your left, from 2226 to 2238 Silver Lake Blvd.

Continue alongside the reservoir for just under 0.5 mile. After crossing Rockford Road, retrace your steps from earlier for a couple of short blocks before turning left

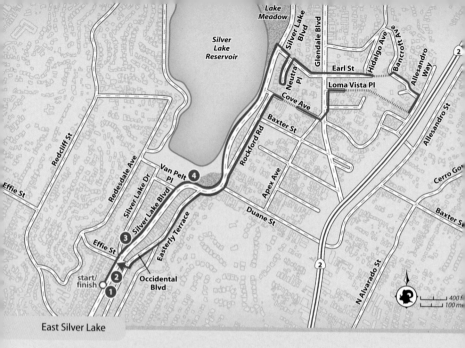

East Silver Lake

Points of Interest

1. **Yolk** 1626 Silver Lake Blvd., Los Angeles, CA 90026; 323-660-4315, shopyolk.com
2. **LA Mill** 1636 Silver Lake Blvd., Los Angeles, CA 90026; 323-663-4441, lamillcoffee.com
3. **The Satellite** 1717 Silver Lake Blvd., Los Angeles, CA 90026; 323-661-4380, thesatellitela.com
4. **Silver Lake Recreation Center** 1850 Silver Lake Blvd., Los Angeles, CA 90026; 323-644-3946

on Easterly Terrace and leaving the noisy boulevard behind. Easterly Terrace is an elevated residential street that runs roughly parallel to Silver Lake Boulevard. Large homes sit high above on the steep hill to your left, some teetering on stilts.

When you reach the fork in the road at Occidental Boulevard, go right to head downhill on Occidental.

Turn right on Effie Street. There's no sign, but it's the first cross street you come to on Occidental Boulevard.

Follow Effie one short block to your starting point at Silver Lake Boulevard.

Echo Park's picturesque lake

26 Echo Park and Angelino Heights

BOUNDARIES: Alvarado St., Sunset Blvd., Bellevue Ave.
DISTANCE: About 2 miles
DIFFICULTY: Moderate (includes stairways)
PARKING: Free street parking is available on Clinton St. Please pay attention to posted signs.

Immediately northwest of downtown LA, this hilly district features some gorgeous homes, many with excellent views, and is convenient to many of the modish shopping and dining destinations that have popped up in the area, particularly along Sunset and Silver Lake Boulevards. Echo Park itself is also a draw; its picturesque lake is a convenient community gathering place and a distinctive focal point. Perhaps the most fascinating features of this neighborhood—the gorgeous Victorian homes of Angelino Heights—stand on a hill just east of Echo Park Lake.

Walk Description

Begin at the intersection of Clinton Street and Belmont Avenue, where Clinton Street ends east of Alvarado Street. Turn right to head south on Belmont. You'll pass a stairway at the end of Clinton, which leads down toward Echo Park Lake.

At the intersection of Bellevue Avenue, turn left to follow the sidewalk that takes you to the steps leading down to Glendale Boulevard. The walkway, formerly marred by graffiti and litter, is nicely trimmed with bougainvillea and palm trees. Cross Glendale Boulevard at the bottom of the steps.

Once across the street, follow the pathway on your left down into ❶ **Echo Park,** and then bear right to continue on the path along the south end of the lake. Echo Park is a vibrant and scenic community center with a heavy Latino cultural influence; you

Back Story: LA's Victorian Suburb

Before it was declared LA's very first Historic Preservation Overlay Zone in 1983, Angelino Heights had survived boom and bust. Developers William W. Stilson and Everett E. Hall created this residential subdivision in 1886 as one of the city's first suburbs—a unique housing tract composed of ornate Queen Anne and Eastlake Victorian homes that was conveniently located on the outskirts of the then-bustling downtown area. Unfortunately, a banking recession in 1888 put a stop to the development, leaving about 50 of these amazing homes to admire today; most of them are concentrated on Carroll and Kellam Avenues. The 1300 block of Carroll Avenue is listed on the National Register of Historic Places for its heavy concentration of Victorians, most of which have been lovingly restored and maintained by the current owners.

Kensington Road, which borders this timeless Victorian oasis, came to be populated with distinguished Craftsman houses during a second wave of development in the early 1900s. As a result, Angelino Heights now offers a rare selection of finely constructed, beautiful homes and a combination of architectural styles not found elsewhere in Los Angeles.

may see a *paleta* (ice pop) salesman circling the lake with his cart. Mothers push strollers along the path, as kids take the paddleboats out for a ride and older gentlemen cast fishing lines out into the placid green water. At the far end of the lake, several jets of water spray high into the air. Continue to follow the path up the east side of the lake, parallel to Echo Park Avenue.

When you reach the paddleboat rental area, about halfway up the east side of the lake, follow the stairs on your right out of the park, and cross Echo Park Avenue at the crosswalk.

Continue on Laguna Avenue, heading northeast, and pass a church on your left. This is a modest residential street populated mostly by older apartment buildings.

Ascend the Crosby Place stairway on your right (opposite 867 Laguna Ave.). The concrete steps are heavily coated in graffiti and bordered by overgrowth, but this vantage point affords a great view of the lake behind you. At the top of the steps, continue straight on Crosby Place. A striking gray Colonial Revival duplex sits on the southwest corner of Crosby Place and West Kensington Road. This is the first of many architecturally fascinating homes you will encounter as you continue on your walk through Angelino Heights.

Turn left on West Kensington Road. Another charming Colonial Revival home sits at 1005 W. Kensington. In stark contrast, a deep-orange, Spanish-style apartment building with a cactus garden in the front is right next door. Continue on West Kensington Road as it curves to the right, crossing Laveta Terrace. The houses on this street become larger and more elaborate as you head farther uphill; many of the Craftsmans date back to the early 1900s. The first Victorian you encounter, at 892 W. Kensington Road, looks incongruous among the many Craftsman and Colonial Revival homes.

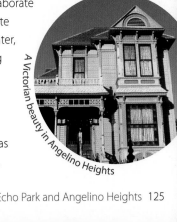

A Victorian beauty in Angelino Heights

Turn right on Douglas Street and continue about two blocks to Edgeware Road. A somber Victorian, heavily shrouded by trees, on the southwest corner of Douglas and West Edgeware, has the look of a haunted house.

Turn left on East Edgeware Road. This street features a few historical Craftsman and Colonial Revival homes scattered among the mostly run-down apartment buildings that were built later in the 20th century. As the road curves south, a view of the nearby downtown skyscrapers opens up ahead.

Turn right on Carroll Avenue, where you'll be transported into another era. Developed as a suburban housing tract for downtown professionals in the 1880s, the Queen Anne and Eastlake Victorian homes along the 1300 block of Carroll have been immaculately restored and maintained thanks to a devoted preservation effort, and they're now listed on the National Register of Historic Places. The juxtaposition of these intricately ornamented homes and the sleek downtown high-rises that lie immediately beyond is a sight to see. This street makes an excellent Halloween destination, as nearly all of the residents get into the spirit by decking out their old-fashioned homes with giant spider webs and hanging dummies. It makes sense, after all, that Michael Jackson's "Thriller" music video was filmed here, at 1345 Carroll Ave.

At the end of Carroll Avenue, turn left on West Edgeware Road, where the quality and maintenance of the residences become more quaint. Head downhill toward noisy US 101.

Turn right on Bellevue Avenue, which runs parallel to the freeway. You also pass Echo Park Lake again, on your right.

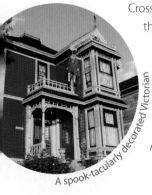

Cross Glendale Boulevard at the signal, and then turn right on the other side to head toward the Clinton Street stairway you passed at the start of your walk. This is the second of three stairways along this block (the first was the Bellevue Avenue stairway you descended earlier).

Ascend the Clinton Street steps, a double stairway that leads back to the junction of Clinton Street and Belmont Avenue, where you began your journey.

A spook-tacularly decorated Victorian

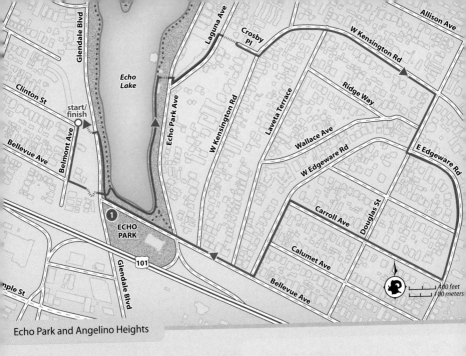

Point of Interest

1 **Echo Park and Echo Park Lake** 751 Echo Park Ave., Los Angeles, CA 90026; 213-847-0929

A view of downtown LA from Elysian Park

27 Elysian Heights

BOUNDARIES: Echo Park Ave., Baxter St., Park Dr., Scott Ave.
DISTANCE: About 0.75 mile
DIFFICULTY: Moderate (includes stairways)
PARKING: Free street parking is available on Baxter St.

Founded in 1886, Elysian Park is LA's second-largest urban oasis (after Griffith Park). Its 600 acres are planted with native chaparral as well as eucalyptus and ficus trees. The park, which is home to Dodger Stadium, also features hiking trails, picnic areas, and playing fields for the nature-craving residents of central and eastern Los Angeles. The hilly area of Elysian Heights, part of the Echo Park neighborhood, abuts the western border of the park, thus providing a delightful escape for residents who wish to forget for a little while that they live in one of the nation's most concrete-bound cities.

Walk Description

Begin at the intersection of Valentine Street and Baxter Street (east of Echo Park Avenue), and head east toward the hill. An elementary school is on your right. This is a peaceful residential neighborhood; the cute, cottagelike homes on the left side of the street are lushly landscaped with assorted plant life, including fruit trees, cactus, and colorful flowers.

Turn right on Avon Street. Ascend the steps on your left, a very long, zigzagging stairway that appears to be carefully maintained—there are even street lights installed alongside the steps. On the hill above are a few modern homes. Pause every once in a while to admire the stunning view behind you, which stretches from Century City to Griffith Park.

Turn right at the top of the stairs onto Park Drive. Directly across the street is ❶ **Elysian Park,** a lush green basin with dirt paths winding down to the bottom. This 600-acre park features an arboretum, countless dirt hiking paths, and picnic areas. Through the eucalyptus trees to the southeast, you can catch an excellent view of downtown. Joggers and dog walkers travel the dirt path just a few yards below, and if you're so inclined, you can hop down the short slope and join them in exploring this big, rustic oasis.

Continue along Park Drive to Duane Street and turn right. Duane has the feel of a narrow country lane as it curves downhill to the left and becomes Avon Street.

Turn right on Lucretia Avenue. Just after the road curves to the left, look for a narrow sidewalk on your right; follow it to the next stairway, nearly as long as the one you ascended earlier, which zigzags down to Avalon Street. As you descend, admire more fabulous views all the way to the coast (on a clear day) to the west, and to the San Gabriel Mountains to the northeast.

Continue straight on Avalon Street one block to Echo Park Avenue.

Turn right on Echo Park Avenue. The next few blocks are considerably less idyllic than the elevated portion of this walk; some of the houses are run-down, and the commercial options don't extend much beyond a liquor store and a hair salon.

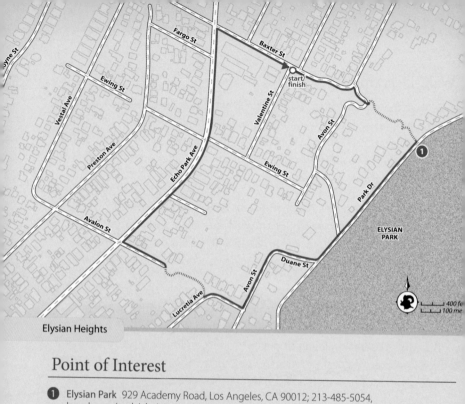

Elysian Heights

Point of Interest

1 Elysian Park 929 Academy Road, Los Angeles, CA 90012; 213-485-5054, laparks.org/park/elysian

When you reach the elementary school near your starting point, turn right on Baxter Street and follow it back to the intersection with Valentine Street, where you began.

A verdant stretch of the Los Angeles River

28 Frogtown (Elysian Valley)

BOUNDARIES: Los Angeles River, CA 2, I-5
DISTANCE: About 1.25 miles
DIFFICULTY: Easy
PARKING: Free parking is available at Marsh Park.

Frogtown is the unofficial name of the formerly scrappy, currently up-and-coming neighborhood sandwiched between the Los Angeles River and I-5 north of CA 110. Officially known as Elysian Valley, this area used to be part of the greater Chavez Ravine community before the construction of Dodger Stadium in 1962. The area is now relatively isolated from the surrounding neighborhoods of Elysian Park, Echo Park, Silver Lake, and Atwater Village by freeways and by the river itself, which has led residents to develop their own distinctive identity, largely inspired by artists and conservationists involved with the LA River's restoration.

In 2014, the nonprofit Friends of the Los Angeles River (FoLAR) opened The Frog Spot, a convenient way station where cyclists riding the popular bike path alongside the river can stop for free ice water and reasonably priced snacks and ice pops. The Frog Spot welcomes noncyclists as well, with free Wi-Fi, maps of the river, docent-led river walks, yoga classes, and live music. It's open only on weekends in the summer, though, so time your visit accordingly if you want to check it out.

Walk Description

Begin in the parking lot for ❶ **Marsh Park,** a beautifully (and drought consciously) designed community park that was expanded in recent years to include a grassy play meadow, a nature trail, and kinetic exercise stations. Plan to spend some time exploring the park, admiring the gorgeous Spanish mission–inspired picnic pavilion and thoughtful landscape design, and maybe even getting in a little workout. (This is also a great spot to use the restroom, as portable toilets are the only option elsewhere on this route, at least as of this writing.) Make your way north through the park, past the restrooms and picnic area to exit through the decorative gate leading out to the Los Angeles River Greenway Trail.

Turn right to follow the path, staying right to make way for cyclists. To your left, the concrete channel wall slopes down to the water. This stretch of the LA River, known as the Glendale Narrows, is a soft-bottomed channel with especially lush flora. It's a popular stretch for fishing, bird-watching, and even kayaking. If you squint your way past the surrounding concrete, you could almost believe you were on the banks of an unadulterated natural waterway as opposed to a paved flood channel in the middle of the city. This is also a particularly pleasant section of the bike/pedestrian path, as it's shaded by the sycamores that border Marsh Park. Continue walking past a skate park and a shady pocket park adjacent to Marsh that features colorful play sculptures of a rattlesnake, frog, and turtle.

After walking along the path for about a third of a mile, you'll come to ❷ **Spoke Bicycle Cafe,** a bike-rental/repair shop with a coffee cart and ample comfortable seating. At the time of this writing, Spoke was still in a state of expansion but already has an undeniably hip and artistic feel, with colorful mural art, a fire pit, vintage tchotchkes, repurposed wood furnishings, and lots of liberally tattooed patrons. It's a strong indicator of things to come—this up-and-coming stretch along the river feels like it's very much on the precipice of exploding into one of northeast LA's coolest destinations, with at least some level of gentrification no doubt following on the heels of the growing independent artist community.

After checking out Spoke, return to the pathway and walk another third of a mile, passing another sycamore-shaded green space known as Elysian Valley Gateway Park.

After just under another third of a mile, you'll come upon ❸ The Frog Spot (assuming you visit on a summer weekend). Whereas Spoke feels a little edgy and oriented toward locals, The Frog Spot is bright, friendly, and welcoming, luring in cyclists with the promise of ice-cold cucumber water and offering a steady schedule of free public programs during the summer, including the aforementioned yoga classes, live concerts, and nature walks. Wine and beer are served on Saturdays after 2 p.m., and there's a bocce court and bike-repair stand. This is the final destination of your walk, so after enjoying a cup of coffee, snack, and/or refreshing beverage, turn around and retrace your steps (again, yielding to cyclists) to Marsh Park along the Los Angeles River Greenway Trail, this time enjoying views of Glendale's Forest Lawn Memorial Park and the San Gabriel Mountains to the north.

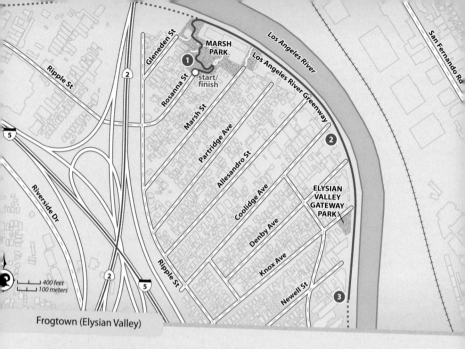

400 feet
100 meters

Frogtown (Elysian Valley)

Points of Interest

1 **Marsh Park** 2944 Gleneden St., Los Angeles, CA 90039; 310-589-3200, tinyurl.com/marshparkla

2 **Spoke Bicycle Cafe** 3050 N. Coolidge St., Los Angeles, CA 90039; 323-684-1130, spokebicyclecafe.com

3 **The Frog Spot** 2825 Benedict St., Los Angeles, CA 90039; 323-223-0585, folar.org/frogspot

29 El Pueblo de Los Angeles and Chinatown

BOUNDARIES: US 101, Alameda St., CA 110
DISTANCE: About 2 miles
DIFFICULTY: Easy
PARKING: There are paid parking lots on Alameda and Los Angeles Sts. There is also limited metered parking on Alameda, across from Union Station, as well as on surrounding side streets, but it's easiest to take the Metro public rail system to this walk. After all, it does begin at the hub of LA's (admittedly limited) subway system.
NEAREST METRO STATION: Union Station, 800 N. Alameda St.

This walk is about as diverse as it gets, exploring both El Pueblo de Los Angeles, home to the area's first settlers, and Chinatown, which is a thriving hub for the city's Chinese American community and a standard tourist attraction. Both neighborhoods now serve as enduring tributes to the history of the settlers and immigrants who have contributed to the development of the greater Los Angeles multicultural society. Your journey begins at one of the city's most recognizable Art Deco landmarks and its central hub for public transit, Union Station.

Walk Description

Begin at ❶ **Union Station** at 800 N. Alameda St. This wonderfully romantic building, opened in 1939, combines the influence of Art Deco and Spanish Colonial Revival architecture to splendid effect. If you traveled here by car, walk through the colossal arched entryway and spend a few minutes taking in the gorgeous painted ceilings, intricate inlaid marble floors and walls, ornate black iron chandeliers, and historic Art Deco furnishings of America's "last great rail station." On the north side of the station is an enclosed patio with a colorful tiled wall fountain. Union Station's resident upscale eatery, Traxx restaurant and bar, offers alfresco dining on this patio.

After you finish exploring the station, exit through the south doorway, and walk across the brick-paved plaza to the Metropolitan Water District building to admire the lovely circular fountain out front, which is tiled in a brilliant fish-scale design. Return to the plaza, and head west toward Alameda Street.

Follow Los Angeles Street across Alameda to enter El Pueblo de Los Angeles, the approximate site of the original town founded by settlers in 1781, back when California still belonged to Mexico. You'll pass the grassy area known as Father Serra Park, which features a statue of the beloved Franciscan priest.

Continue straight along the pedestrian walkway Paseo de la Plaza. As you approach the gathering center of the plaza—an enormous gazebo that acts as a stage for mariachi bands and street performers—you pass the Biscailuz Building on your right. This former home of the Mexican Consulate General now houses the Mexican Cultural Institute. A vibrant mural by Leo Politi, *Blessing of the Animals,* graces one wall of the building.

Head south across the plaza to check out some of El Pueblo's historic buildings. At the corner of Main Street and Arcadia Street are the Masonic Hall (established in 1858); Los Angeles' first theatrical house, the Merced Theatre (established 1870); and the Pico House, an extravagant Italianate luxury

Union Station entrance

hotel commissioned by the last governor of Mexican California, Pío Pico, in 1870. Los Angeles' first fire station, the ❷ Old Plaza Firehouse (established in 1884), sits at the southeast corner of the plaza; the onetime home of Engine Company No. 1, the restored building is now a museum for late-19th-century firefighting memorabilia (free tours are available). There's also the Chinese American Museum and, across Main Street to the northeast, La Plaza de Cultura y Artes, a museum dedicated to the Mexican American in Southern California.

Walk northeast back across the plaza and look for the entrance to Olvera Street, which is identified by a large brown cross. The rich aroma of leather emanates from the purse-and-belt-vendor stalls that crowd the entrance. This one-block pedestrian alley is a popular tourist attraction designed to re-create the type of thriving marketplace you might find in Tijuana or Ensenada, Mexico. At 10 Olvera St., you come to the ❸ Avila Adobe, the oldest existing house in Los Angeles, built by Don Francisco Avila in 1818 (free tours are available). As you continue through the alley, you pass an eclectic mix of stalls and shops selling souvenirs, Western clothing, jewelry, Mexican artwork, candies, *pan dulce,* and other treats. The ❹ América Tropical Interpretive Center, at 125 Paseo de la Plaza, is dedicated to the once controversial and whitewashed mural by David Alfaro Siqueiros. If you prefer to skip the snack-food stalls and sit down for a full, authentic Mexican meal, ❺ Casa La Golondrina, at 17 Olvera St., is not only a popular spot but also one of the oldest Mexican restaurants in the city.

You emerge from Olvera Street onto Cesar E. Chavez Avenue. Turn left here.

In less than a block, turn right on Main Street, and follow it to where Main merges with Alameda Street.

Turn left on Alameda, and then immediately turn left again onto Ord Street. ❻ Philippe the Original occupies the northwest corner of this intersection. Even if you don't plan to eat at the legendary deli and French-dip emporium, you ought to step inside to check out the joint's singular ambience. The interior appears to have changed little since it was established in 1908: sawdust covers the floors, and long communal picnic tables lined with benches occupy most of the space.

Back Story: A Tale of Two Neighborhoods

Interestingly enough, both El Pueblo de Los Angeles and Chinatown have been moved from their original sites. The actual location where Mexican settlers established their village in 1781 was closer to the Los Angeles River, just east of where Union Station stands today, but flooding in 1818 forced them to move to higher ground—the current site of El Pueblo. The original neighborhood known as Chinatown was rudely displaced to make way for construction of Union Station in the 1930s. The Chinese immigrants eventually developed the thriving community a few blocks northwest in what is now more appropriately referred to as New Chinatown.

The building is huge, offering private booth seating in the rear of the first floor and several private rooms upstairs. In addition to the legendary sandwich, you can purchase all manner of deli items behind the busy counter, as well as Philippe's famous 9¢ cup of coffee. Public restrooms are also available here.

Exit back onto Ord Street, and turn right to continue west three short blocks to Broadway. Notice the Little Jewel of New Orleans, a Big Easy–based deli and grocer.

Turn right on Broadway, staying on the east side of the street; you're now on Chinatown's main drag. As you head north on Broadway, you pass jewelry and clothing stores, a pungent fish market, and several tiny shops selling Chinese dried goods and spices.

Cross Alpine Street, and arrive at the 800 block of Broadway, which is home to three shopping malls: Dynasty Center, Chinatown Plaza, and ❼ **Saigon Plaza.** The plaza most worth poking your head into is Saigon, an outdoor collection of vendor stalls selling clothing, shoes, slippers, and a delectable array of deep-fried treats.

When you reach College Street, cross to the west side of Broadway, and continue north. You pass a beautiful tiled mural next door to the Plum Tree Inn restaurant, at 913 Broadway.

Pass the first gateway you come to, which leads into an alley, and continue to the East Gate, the magnificent entryway to Chinatown's Central Plaza. The colorful wooden portal is an example of Neo-Chinese architecture, which is carried through in the gorgeous tile work and gaily painted balconies inside the plaza.

Turn left to enter through the East Gate, following Gin Ling Way into the Central Plaza. The Wonder Food Bakery is just inside the entrance on your left, and a lovely fountain trickles on your right. Gin Ling Way is hung with red and white paper lanterns and lined with touristy shops selling a variety of Chinese tchotchkes. On your left, just before Mei Ling Way, you pass a massive wishing-well sculpture that dates to 1939; toss your coins toward little signs representing Health, Money, Love, and other good fortunes. As you cross Mei Ling Way, look left to see the five-tier pagoda atop ❽ **Hop Louie,** a distinctive Chinatown landmark constructed in 1941. A restaurant and lounge from its inception, Hop Louie closed its kitchen in late 2016, but the bar—its real drawing card—remains open.

Cross Hill Street, and continue into Chinatown's West Plaza by way of Chung King Court. Chung King Court dead-ends at Chung King Road, another pedestrian walkway that has attracted a spate of artists in recent years, making the West Plaza a destination for hot new gallery openings.

Turn left on Chung King Road to explore some of the galleries before returning to Chung King Court.

Exit West Plaza by way of Chung King Court and turn right on Hill Street to head south. If you've managed to hold out this long, ❾ **Foo Chow Restaurant,** on the southwest corner of Chung King Court and Hill Street, is an excellent place to stop for a generous helping of noodles, seafood, or moo-shu for not a lot of money; it was also a filming location for the hit action comedy *Rush Hour.*

Cross College Street and continue south on Hill Street, admiring the view of the downtown skyline straight ahead. At 825 Hill St. is the Chinese United Methodist Church; appropriately enough, this house of worship incorporates elements of both Chinese- and Western-style architecture.

Turn left on Alpine Street and continue one block back to Broadway.

Turn right on Broadway, but this time remain on the west side of the street. Cathay Bank, the first Chinese American–owned bank in Southern California, sits on the southwest corner of Alpine and Broadway. Continue south on Broadway, passing the ❿ **Far East Plaza** on your right. This shopping mall has become a hot spot for noted food in the city: Chego, Scoops ice cream, and Howlin Ray's, to name a few.

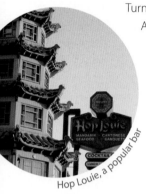

Hop Louie, a popular bar

Turn left on Ord Street, retracing your steps a few blocks back to Alameda Street.

Turn right on Alameda. On the east side of the street, at 900 N. Alameda, look for the imposing Mission/Spanish Revival facade of the US Post Office Terminal Annex, which was designed by Gilbert S. Underwood in 1938.

Cross Cesar E. Chavez Avenue to return to your starting point at Union Station.

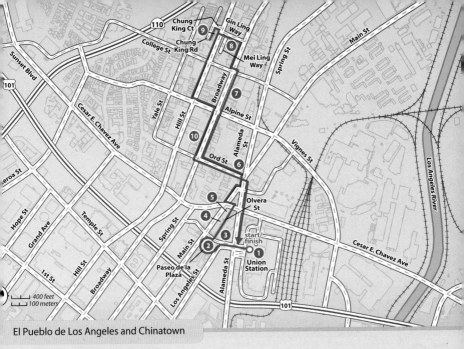

El Pueblo de Los Angeles and Chinatown

Points of Interest

1 Union Station 800 N. Alameda St., Los Angeles, CA 90012; metro.net/about/union-station

2 Old Plaza Firehouse 501 N. Los Angeles St., Los Angeles, CA 90012; 213-485-8437

3 Avila Adobe 10 Olvera St., Los Angeles, CA 90012; 213-628-1274

4 América Tropical Interpretive Center 125 Paseo De La Plaza, Los Angeles, CA 90012; 213-628-1274, theamericatropical.org

5 Casa La Golondrina 17 Olvera St., Los Angeles, CA 90012; 213-628-4349

6 Philippe the Original 1001 N. Alameda St., Los Angeles, CA 90012; 213-628-3781, philippes.com

7 Saigon Plaza 800 N. Broadway, Los Angeles, CA 90012

8 Hop Louie 950 Mei Ling Way (inside Central Plaza), Los Angeles, CA 90012; 213-628-4244

9 Foo Chow Restaurant 949 N. Hill St., Los Angeles, CA 90012; 213-485-1294

10 Far East Plaza 727 N. Broadway, Los Angeles, CA 90012

The stunning Walt Disney Concert Hall is the centerpiece of the Music Center complex.

30 Downtown Civic Center

BOUNDARIES: US 101, Hope St., Main St., Fourth St.
DISTANCE: About 2 miles
DIFFICULTY: Moderate (includes stairways)
PARKING: Like every building downtown, the Cathedral of Our Lady of Angels, where this route begins, requires that you pay for parking. Your best bet is to do this walk on a weekend or on a weekday after 4 p.m., when you can park for a fairly reasonable flat fee. If you attend Sunday Mass, you can park for 3 hours at no charge. Alternatively, you can take the Metro Red Line to the Civic Center stop and walk a block north to your starting point at the cathedral. Alternatively, you can always try your luck with metered parking on the surrounding streets.
NEAREST METRO STATION: Civic Center, First St. and Hill St. (Red Line)

The Civic Center, as the area of downtown just south of US 101 and just east of CA 110 is called, has been subject to a flurry of development over the past few years as part of a revitalization effort, and the overhaul is far from over. Parking structures have been leveled to make way for more commercial, residential, retail, and hotel space. Presently, the effect of all this expansion is occasionally successful, as in the case of the majestic Walt Disney

Concert Hall. At other times, it's discordant: witness the decidedly ungraceful design of the Cathedral of Our Lady of Angels. This walk explores these new additions to the downtown cityscape, as well as the institutions that form the city's historic core, such as City Hall and Grand Central Market.

Walk Description

Begin at the ❶ **Cathedral of Our Lady of Angels,** at 555 W. Temple St. Regardless of whether you park in the structure or walk from the Metro station, enter the cathedral grounds via the lower courtyard, which is graced with a waterfall fountain. Ascend the stairs into the main courtyard to access the cathedral itself, as well as a little café and gift shop. Before proceeding toward the church, wander to the northeast corner of the upper courtyard, where you'll discover an interesting sculpture garden featuring an assortment of wild and domestic creatures. The cathedral looms formidably ahead. Architect Rafael Moneo constructed the massive edifice out of adobe-colored concrete, creating an oddly striated effect with his layered formation of the outer walls. For more architecture, gaze across the freeway: that's the Ramón C. Cortines School of Visual and Performing Arts, perhaps one of the most uniquely designed public high school campuses in the city.

Enter the cathedral by way of the great bronze doors on the left side of the facade. The starkly modern interior feels refreshingly cool on hot days and carries through the exterior theme of neutral tones in stone, wood, and marble. Filtered sunlight enters through the gray-tinted Spanish alabaster windows. Take a few moments to explore, sticking to the perimeter of the building if there is a service under way, and you'll find a collection of sculptures and framed oil paintings that are dwarfed by the dimensions of the interior space. The most striking pieces of art are the hand-painted tapestries lining the walls of the inner sanctuary; they portray a sampling of the Roman Catholic community—people young and old of various ethnicities. (The cathedral offers free group tours.)

After exploring the cathedral, exit back into the plaza the same way you came in, return to street level, and turn right to head west along Temple Street.

Cross Grand Avenue and then cross to the south side of Temple so that you're on the southwest corner of the intersection. Ascend the stairs to reach the collection of theaters that make up the ❷ **Music Center** complex.

Turn left at the top of the stairs to walk through the Los Angeles Times Garden Courtyard, a paved walkway, complete with tables and chairs, between towering concrete columns. On your right is the Ahmanson Theatre and then the Mark Taper Forum, a striking cylindrical theater decorated with an abstract bas-relief. Note that there are public restrooms on your left.

After passing the reflecting pools that front the Mark Taper, you emerge into the main courtyard of the Music Center; the classy outdoor Pinot Grill operates in the evenings here. The centerpiece of the plaza is an elevated dancing fountain built around an expressive and semireligious sculpture titled *Peace on Earth*. This large monument was dedicated by artist Jacques Lipchitz in 1969 as "a symbol of peace to the peoples of the world," according to the inscription at the base of the fountain. Take a few minutes to enjoy your vantage point in the midst of the Music Center complex. To the northwest, you can see the glass-and-steel Department of Water and Power building, flanked by its own magnificent high-spouting fountains. The distinctive City Hall tower (established in 1929), which incorporates classical and Art Deco design elements to elegant effect, rises beyond Grand Park directly southeast.

Before descending the stairway to Grand Avenue on the east side of the fountain, take a second to admire the metal sculpture of an open doorway by Robert Graham. The piece, called *Dance Door*, features a bas-relief of nude dancers reminiscent of Edgar Degas's ballerinas.

At the bottom of the stairs, turn right on Grand. Pass the county courthouse on your left just before reaching First Street, at which point the burnished, mellifluous wings of Frank Gehry's Walt Disney Concert Hall come into view. Also part of the Music Center, this world-renowned architectural masterpiece is now the permanent home of the Los Angeles Philharmonic. (For information about tours of Disney Hall, call 213-972-4399.)

Cross First Street, and enter the lobby through the glass doors on the east side of the building (facing Grand Avenue). The lobby is a study in curved surfaces: white-painted walls and ceilings with blond wood finishing. This is a tourist spot, so you'll find another gift shop and café here. Self-guided audio tours of the architectural highlights of the concert hall are available for a small fee.

Exit Disney Hall back onto Grand Avenue, and then turn left to backtrack slightly to the corner of First Street. Turn left on First Street, remaining on the same side of the street as the concert hall.

Continue northwest on First for almost one block. Just before you reach Hope Street, turn left to follow the stairway up to the Music Center's Blue Ribbon Garden, hidden behind the concert hall. This lovely 1-acre park offers plentiful shade trees and places to rest. Continue walking through the park to its centerpiece: a gently burbling sculpture fountain in the shape of a giant rose. The sculpture, covered in a mosaic of blue-and-white china pieces, was designed by Frank Gehry as a tribute to Walt Disney's wife, Lillian Bounds Disney, on behalf of her children and grandchildren.

Proceed toward the far end of the park, and then turn left to cut through the charming outdoor Children's Amphitheatre. Descend the stairway back down to Grand Avenue and turn right.

Cross Second Street and you'll be standing in front of ❸ **The Broad** museum, which houses the modern-art collection of Eli and Edythe Broad, noted LA philan-thropists. Opened in 2015, the museum charges no admission but requires reser-vations when busy. Continue straight, past a grassy courtyard with an outdoor coffee bar and restaurant in the back; then cross Grand Avenue at Third Street and turn left to backtrack down Grand a couple hundred feet to the entrance of the ❹ **Museum of Contemporary Art (MOCA).**

Turn right to enter MOCA's outdoor plaza, which is identified by a sculptural bloom of airplane parts by Nancy Rubins.

Turn right to follow the narrow courtyard built around a long strip of reflecting pool and shaded by magnolia trees, passing the Omni Hotel on your left. As the plaza opens, you'll find yourself overlooking the spectacular Watercourt fountain, which doubles as a stage for free outdoor concerts during the summer. (Visit grandperformances.org for more information.)

Descend either the escalator or the stairway to your right, which deposits you in a covered hallway of numerous lunch-hour spots for the suit-and-tie crowd. You can grab a bite here, but you'd be better off choosing something more interesting from the variety at the Grand Central Market, which you will reach shortly. Turn right to emerge into the light on the same level as the Watercourt fountain.

Walk around the front of the Watercourt, and then look for the stairway on your right that leads to the park below. Descend the first set of steps, and then continue down the next long stairway, which runs parallel to the sometimes-operational Angels Flight funicular. The sloping grassy park on your right is home to the bench looking over the city from the movie *500 Days of Summer*.

At the bottom of the stairs, cross Hill Street to reach the entrance of ❺ **Grand Central Market**, LA's famous open-air market, open seven days a week. Founded in 1917, it hasn't lost its charm or the public's interest. You'll find plenty of tempting lunch ideas here. Walk all the way through the market until you emerge onto Broadway.

Turn left on Broadway. At the southeast corner of Broadway and Third Street is the ❻ **Bradbury Building**, designed by George H. Wyman in the 1890s. You must check out the inside of this architectural landmark, which is open to the public; the interior is illuminated by natural light filtering through the translucent domed roof high above the atrium. The elaborate stairways are composed of cast iron in an eclectic Victorian design. You may recognize the distinctive surroundings from the climactic fight scene in *Blade Runner*.

Return to the street and continue northeast along Broadway. This part of downtown represents a different era, but it offers its share of interesting sites. For example, you'll notice the delightfully tacky Guadalupe Wedding Chapel, its Romanesque facade ornamented with faux Corinthian columns—very

GRAND CENTRAL MARKET
SINCE 1917
Grand Central Market

Vegas—on the west side of the street just after you cross Third. As you approach Second Street, check out the *Los Angeles Times* parking structure on your right, which features an elaborate bas-relief artwork depicting a stylized history of California's colonization.

Turn right on Second Street. The LAPD headquarters is on your left, and to your right when crossing the alley is The Edison, a large, popular 1920s-themed bar that resides in an old power substation. **7 Pitfire Pizza Company,** a very good bet for a lunch of fresh salads and mouthwatering pizza and panini, is on the southeast corner of Second and Main Streets. Across from there, at 114 E. Second St., is St. Vibiana's Cathedral, dedicated in 1876. The cathedral has been damaged by an earthquake and threatened with demolition in the last century, but it still stands today as the result of passionate preservation efforts.

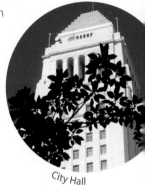

City Hall

Turn left on Main Street. The Caltrans headquarters is on your right. The extraordinary (and imposing) glass-and-steel building occupies an entire block and was designed by prestigious architect Thom Mayne. An enormous *1-0-0* looms above the street, marking the building's address on Main Street.

Cross First Street and proceed to the public entrance to **8 City Hall,** on your left below the pedestrian bridge that connects to City Hall East. (If it's a weekend or holiday, City Hall is closed to the public. In that case, turn left and walk through the lawn in front of City Hall to admire the architecture.) The attractive Art Deco building is distinguished by its white tower; the concrete used for its construction is said to have been made from sand taken from each of California's 58 counties. Enter the building, get a visitor's badge from security, and take the elevator to the third floor, where you can admire the gorgeous inlaid marble floor and the tile ceilings of the rotunda. Next, take the elevator up to the observation deck on the 27th floor, where you can admire 360-degree views of the city. After taking in the vista, return to ground level, and exit where you entered. Head back toward First Street, and hang a right to go through City Hall's shaded lawn.

Turn right on Spring Street toward the pedestrian crossing, and cross into
⑨ **Grand Park.** Dubbed "the park for everyone," Grand Park is a 12-acre public
space that spans three blocks. Picnicking, festivals, and major city celebrations
are held here. Parts of the park were most recently a parking lot, but the area
now includes drought-tolerant gardens, shade trees, hot-pink lawn furniture, and
a whimsical playground.

Walk through the pleasant park, crossing both Broadway and Hill. The last section
runs between a county courthouse and the Hall of Administration, which is essen-
tially the City Hall for county operations. Continue through the park. At the far
end, a magnificent circular fountain projects a refreshing mist over the surrounding benches—a lovely place to take one last break before the end of the walk.

On the other side of the fountain, ascend the stairs back up to Grand Avenue, and
turn right.

Continue half a block to Temple Street, and turn right to return to your starting
point at the cathedral.

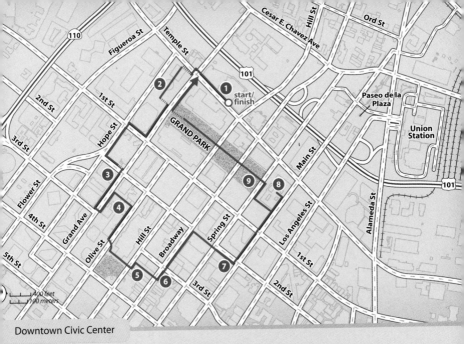

Downtown Civic Center

Points of Interest

① **Cathedral of Our Lady of Angels** 555 W. Temple St., Los Angeles, CA 90012; 213-680-5200, olacathedral.org

② **Music Center (Dorothy Chandler Pavilion, Ahmanson Theatre, Mark Taper Forum, Walt Disney Concert Hall)** 135 N. Grand Ave., Los Angeles, CA 90012; 213-972-7211, musiccenter.org

③ **The Broad** 221 S. Grand Ave., Los Angeles, CA 90012; 213-232-6200, thebroad.org

④ **Museum of Contemporary Art** 250 S. Grand Ave., Los Angeles, CA 90012; 213-626-6222, moca.org

⑤ **Grand Central Market** 317 S. Broadway, Los Angeles, CA 90012; 213-624-2378

⑥ **Bradbury Building** 304 S. Broadway, Los Angeles, CA 90012

⑦ **Pitfire Pizza Company** 108 W. Second St., Los Angeles, CA 90012; 213-808-1200, pitfirepizza.com

⑧ **City Hall** 200 N. Spring St., Los Angeles, CA 90012; 213-473-7001, lacity.org

⑨ **Grand Park** 200 N. Grand Ave., Los Angeles, CA 90012; grandparkla.org

Pershing Square cityscape

31 Downtown Financial and Jewelry Districts

BOUNDARIES: Broadway, Fourth St., Figueroa St., Seventh St.
DISTANCE: About 1.5 miles
DIFFICULTY: Moderate (includes stairways)
PARKING: Metered parking is available on Grand Ave., north of Hope Pl.
NEAREST METRO STATION: Pershing Square, Hill St. between Fourth St. and Fifth St. (Red Line)

At first glance, downtown Los Angeles's Financial District—with its anonymous mirrored-glass skyscrapers that could be from just about any modern metropolis—lacks personality. But take some time to explore what's hidden among all those tall buildings, and you'll discover several of downtown's treasures, such as the innovative architecture of the Central Library, the extravagant interior of the Millennium Biltmore Hotel, and the thoughtfully designed Bunker Hill steps, as well as numerous public art projects. This walk also passes through the busy Jewelry District, home to some of most beautiful movie palaces in the country.

Walk Description

Begin on Grand Avenue between Hope Place and Fifth Street and head southwest, toward Fifth Street.

Turn right on Fifth Street. The stately brick tower of the Millennium Biltmore Hotel rises on the southwest corner of Grand and Fifth Street. Notice the classical Art Deco high-rise known as One Bunker Hill on the northwest corner; this 14-story building, composed of solid limestone and buff-colored terra-cotta, once housed Southern California Edison.

Turn right to ascend the gracefully curving Bunker Hill staircase. An elevated fountain built to resemble a stony brook runs down the center of the wide steps, which are also known as LA's own Spanish Steps. Look behind you to the other side of Fifth Street to see the north entrance of the Central Library; an inscription carved into the stone facade reads, "Books alone are liberal and free: They give to all who ask. They emancipate all who serve them faithfully." As you make your way up the shallow steps, notice the cylindrical Library Tower reaching skyward on your right. Recently downgraded to the second tallest building in LA by the newly constructed Wilshire Grand, this distinctive landmark has been branded with the U.S. Bank logo on its lofty lighthouse—an unfortunate but inevitable sign of the times. The Citigroup building, known informally as the "*LA Law* building," is on your left.

At the top of the steps is a small, circular plaza built around a fountain sculpture of a nude woman in bronze. Continue straight ahead onto Hope Street and notice the gleaming wings of Walt Disney Concert Hall (see previous walk) several blocks northeast.

When you reach the YMCA building on your left, just before Fourth Street, turn left to cut through the outdoor plaza. Various metal sculptures depicting male and female figures in athletic pursuits grace the patio.

As you continue through the plaza, the mirrored-glass cylindrical towers of the ❶ Westin Bonaventure Hotel loom ahead. Follow the first pedestrian walkway you encounter to enter the building; from there, descend the spiral stairway all the way to the lobby. (Or, if you prefer, ride down in one of the building's famous glass elevators so that you can admire the view.) Built in 1978 and the setting of the

'80s sitcom *It's a Living,* the Bonaventure now looks dated inside, with lots of concrete and very little natural light. Once you've reached the lobby, exit the hotel through the glass doors on your left to Flower Street.

Turn right on Flower Street and continue across Fifth Street. Cross to the other side of Flower so that you're on the same side as the ❷ **Central Library.**

Follow the long, stepped walkway leading through Maguire Gardens to the library's entrance, and admire the facade of the 1920s public building, which successfully incorporates elements of modern urban architecture with the ancient influence of Egyptian, Roman, Byzantine, and Islamic civilizations. The library's solitary tower is capped with a colorful tiled pyramid depicting a sunburst and torch to represent the light of knowledge. A tiled reflecting pool runs down the center of the path leading up to the library entrance, and a lovely wall of spouting fountains lies in an alcove off to the right of the main entryway plaza. Cafe Pinot, an upscale restaurant serving California/French cuisine, is to your left. The grassy public space and decorative fountains surrounding the library are known as the Maguire Gardens.

Enter the library through the striking northwest-facing portal. Continue through the dark hallway into the main lobby, which is graced with a vibrantly painted ceiling. LA's Central Library is worth taking some time to explore; of particular architectural interest is the Tom Bradley Wing at the east end of the building, which consists of a dramatic, light-filled, eight-story atrium. You should also head upstairs to admire the Lodwrick M. Cook Rotunda, with its intricately stenciled ceiling and enormous chandelier.

After exploring the interior of the library, return to the main lobby on the first floor, and leave the building through the southwest-facing exit (toward Hope Street).

Once outside, descend the first two sets of stairs and then turn left to follow the sidewalk—don't descend the last set of stairs to street level. On your right is the Hilton Checkers Hotel, a nicely restored 1920s building with ornate molded details.

When you reach Grand Avenue, carefully cross the street and then turn left. When you reach the valet parking area of the ❸ **Millennium Biltmore Hotel,** turn right to proceed to the hotel's rear entrance. This Beaux Arts landmark, which opened for business in 1923, remains one of LA's finest classic hotels. The hotel's lobby is splendid, ornamented with a richly carved and painted ceiling, thick rugs, and distinguished furnishings.

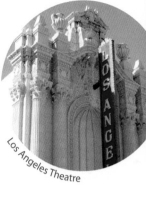

Los Angeles Theatre

Continue straight through the lobby and then turn right into the building's grand hallway, which is lined with intricately carved stone pillars. Turn left at the elevators and descend the stairs into the front lobby. It doesn't seem possible, but this massive, high-ceilinged room—featuring an impressive arched ceiling with an intricate inlaid-wood design and a lovely central fountain—is even more magnificent than the first lobby you entered. Walk through the lobby to exit onto Olive Street.

Cross Olive Street to Pershing Square. Still considered a major downtown landmark, this public park has fallen hard from its former glory as a lush oasis in the center of the city. Today, this mostly concrete-paved space looks outdated, with its colorful geometric walls and sculptures, but it does afford a convenient raised clearing from which to survey the surrounding architecture. Luckily, it's slated for a major makeover. To the northwest is the distinguished brick facade of the Biltmore Hotel you just exited; immediately northeast of the Biltmore is the Gas Company Tower, a dramatic marble-and-steel high-rise with a curved, boatlike glass atrium at the top. Northeast of Pershing Square is the Art Deco–style Title Guarantee and Trust Building, which dates back to 1930. And if you look southwest, you can catch a glimpse of the outdoor clock (colorfully neon-lit at night) that overlooks the patio outside the Oviatt Building penthouse, another Art Deco landmark. At the southwest end of the park, a towering fountain that resembles a giant rain gutter spills a murky stream of water into a shallow, stone-lined pool.

Cross Pershing Square to Hill Street and turn right.

Turn left on Sixth Street and walk one block to Broadway. You're now in downtown's bustling and somewhat seedy Jewelry District.

Back Story: What Ever Happened to Bunker Hill?

Founded in 1867, the area currently referred to as the Financial District sits atop Bunker Hill, a residential neighborhood that was leveled in the 1950s to make way for the skyscrapers that mark downtown Los Angeles today. Once a bustling residential community for Los Angeles professionals and their families, Bunker Hill degenerated over time and eventually became populated with unsavory rooming houses. In the 1960s, LA's Community Redevelopment Agency demolished what was left of the neighborhood's Victorian residences to make way for a "new downtown," complete with shiny skyscrapers, to signal the city's prosperity and status as an international commercial and banking center.

Turn right on Broadway, which is in the infancy of the Bringing Back Broadway movement, a call to bring live theater back to this stretch of downtown. For example, the ornate French Baroque ❹ **Los Angeles Theatre,** at 615 S. Broadway, hasn't been a working movie palace for many years, but it's available for filming and for private rentals. To visit the stunning interior of the theater, contact the Los Angeles Conservancy's Last Remaining Seats program at 213-623-2489.

❺ **Clifton's,** one of LA's last surviving cafeteria-style restaurants, is located at 648 S. Broadway. In business since 1935, the eatery has a Disney–meets– natural-history-museum feel. It was recently revamped into a hip multistory bar and grill that honors its old-school-cafeteria vibe. Clifton's is absolutely worth stopping in for a meal or a piece of pie so that you can marvel at the restaurant's throwback mountain woods–themed interior.

Turn right on Seventh Street and walk to St. Vincent's Court, on your right.

Turn right to explore this charming alley, which features a collection of Middle Eastern delis and bakeries housed behind Parisian café–style facades. Retrace your steps to Seventh Street.

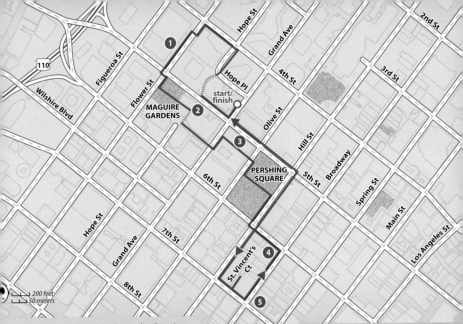

Downtown Financial and Jewelry Districts

Points of Interest

1. **Westin Bonaventure Hotel** 404 S. Figueroa St., Los Angeles, CA 90071; 213-624-1000, westin.com/bonaventure

2. **Central Library** 630 W. Fifth St., Los Angeles, CA 90071; 213-228-7000, lapl.org/central

3. **Millennium Biltmore Hotel** 506 S. Grand Ave., Los Angeles, CA 90071; 213-624-1011, tinyurl.com/millenniumbiltmorela

4. **Los Angeles Theatre** 615 S. Broadway, Los Angeles, CA 90014; 213-629-2939, losangelestheatre.com

5. **Clifton's** 648 S. Broadway, Los Angeles, CA 90014; 213-627-1673, cliftonsla.com

Turn right on Seventh and then turn right on Hill Street, walking for two blocks.

Turn left on Fifth Street and continue two more blocks, passing between the towering edifices of the Biltmore Hotel and the Gas Company Tower.

Turn right on Grand Avenue to return to your starting point.

Festive lanterns greet visitors to Little Tokyo.

32 Little Tokyo

BOUNDARIES: Temple St., Los Angeles St., Third St., Alameda St.
DISTANCE: About 0.75 mile
DIFFICULTY: Easy
PARKING: Metered street parking is available on First St.
NEAREST METRO STATION: Civic Center, First St. and Hill St. (Red Line)

Located in downtown Los Angeles, just south of US 101 and next door to the Arts District, is Little Tokyo, a neighborhood that simultaneously projects multicultural urban cool while retaining its ties to Japanese American history. There's plenty to draw locals and tourists alike, such as authentic Japanese eateries too numerous to count, spas offering affordable Shiatsu treatments, shops selling colorful knickknacks, the Japanese American National Museum, and the Geffen Contemporary extension of the Museum of Contemporary Art (MOCA).

Walk Description

Begin at the intersection of Central Avenue and First Street, where Central Avenue ends and transforms into an open pedestrian plaza. On the east side of the clearing is the site of the ❶ **Japanese American National Museum,** a graceful sandstone, metal, and glass building that was designed by Gyo Obata, who also designed the Air and Space Museum in Washington, DC. Just across the plaza, the museum's National Center for the Preservation of Democracy is housed in a lovely old brick building (with an ultramodern addition) dating from 1925 that originally was the site of the Nishi Hongwanji Buddhist Temple.

Head north through the plaza toward ❷ **The Geffen Contemporary at MOCA,** which houses installations that are too large to fit in the museum's California Plaza location downtown (see Walk 30). After you pass the warehouselike home of MOCA's easternmost satellite, you'll come to the ❸ **Go For Broke Monument,** which commemorates more than 16,000 Japanese American veterans of World War II who voluntarily went to Europe and the Pacific Rim to fight for the same country that sent their families to internment camps back in the States. Surviving veterans occasionally volunteer as guides at the monument, and if you have the time to talk to one of these incredibly brave and patriotic men, you'll no doubt be amazed at the stories he has to tell.

Head back to the intersection of Central and First. On your way, you'll pass a number of items of interest on your right. First is the Aoyama Tree, a Moreton Bay fig tree that was planted in 1920 and marks the former location of one of the oldest Buddhist temples in the city, the Koyasan Daishi Mission. The home of the National Center for the Preservation of Democracy is next, then the ❹ **Go For Broke National Education Center,** where you can learn more about the Japanese American experience during World War II. Lastly, a piece of public art representing Toyo Miyatake's camera. Miyatake was forced into a American concentration camp, to use the parlance of the time, during the war. He sneaked a camera into the internment camp at Manzanar, some 3 hours north, and documented life there.

At the intersection of Central and First, turn right to head west one block on First Street, passing a crowded collection of Japanese sweet shops, sushi restaurants, and popular ramen houses such as Mr. Ramen and Daikokuya. Glance downward along the north side to see Little Tokyo's history engraved in the pavement—this is Little Tokyo's Historic District.

Turn left on San Pedro Street, which is called Judge John Aiso Street in the opposite direction. As you continue southwest, you'll come to the site of Seiji Kunishima's *Stonerise* sculpture, a massive art piece composed of roughly textured black granite blocks that sits in a quiet garden on the north side of the Union Bank building.

At the northwest corner of San Pedro and Second Street is the entrance to Weller Court, also known as Astronaut Ellison S. Onizuka Street, named for the first Japanese American astronaut. This low-key pedestrian street is marked by Shin-kichi Tajiri's *Friendship Knot* sculpture. As you walk through the court, you'll pass Marukai Market, a large grocery store that carries all manner of authentic Japanese goodies. About halfway through the court is a replica of the *Challenger* space shuttle, aboard which Onizuka launched his final space mission.

Walk back to where you entered the court. Cross Second and then cross to the east side of San Pedro Street and turn right to head south. In front of the bank on the southeast corner is a bronze statue of prominent Japanese farmer Sontoku (Kinjiro) Ninomiya, sometimes known as the "peasant sage of Japan."

Before you cross the Azusa Street alley, look up to see a historical marker. You're near the site of the Azusa Street Mission, where the Pentecostal religious movement began. Cross the alley and head into the open plaza, home to the ❺ **Japanese American Cultural and Community Center.** Enter the spacious, brick-paved plaza, designed by Isamu Noguchi. The imposing concrete facade of the center lies directly south.

Enter the center through the massive glass doors and ask if the garden is open. If so, you're in for a treat. The beautiful James Irvine Japanese Garden is a carefully tended paradise that lies in stark contrast to the imposing concrete building that towers above.

Return to ground level and walk back across the plaza to the Azusa Street alley. Follow the short alley through to Second Street.

Cross Second Street and continue through the ❻ **Japanese Village Plaza,** bearing right at the split to continue on the path toward First Street. This mall is the heart of Little Tokyo's shopping district, offering sushi and noodle cafés, shabu-shabu

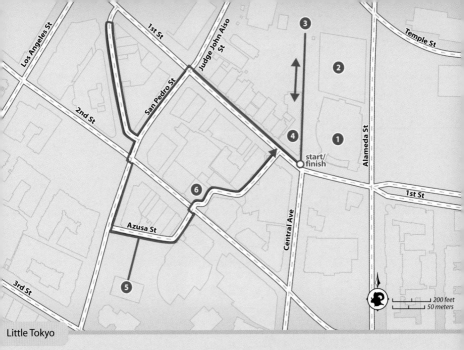

Little Tokyo

Points of Interest

1 Japanese American National Museum/National Center for the Preservation of Democracy
100 N. Central Ave., Los Angeles, CA 90012; 213-625-0414, janm.org

2 The Geffen Contemporary at MOCA   152 N. Central Ave., Los Angeles, CA 90013;
213-625-4390, moca.org/visit/geffen-contemporary

3 Go For Broke Monument   160 N. Central Ave., Los Angeles, CA 90012

4 Go For Broke National Education Center   355 E. First St., Los Angeles, CA 90012;
310-328-0907, goforbroke.org

5 Japanese American Cultural and Community Center/James Irvine Japanese Garden
244 S. San Pedro St., Los Angeles, CA 90012; 213-628-2725, jaccc.org

6 Japanese Village Plaza   335 E. Second St., Los Angeles, CA 90012; japanesevillageplaza.net

dining, knickknack shops, Shiatsu massage, sweets, and plenty of other opportunities to indulge yourself.

After grabbing a snack, meal, or massage in the plaza, exit onto First Street, where you'll find yourself back at your starting point at the intersection of Central Avenue.

An installation at Hauser Wirth & Schimmel

33 Downtown Arts District

BOUNDARIES: E. First St., Santa Fe Ave., Industrial St., Alameda St.
DISTANCE: 2.75 miles
DIFFICULTY: Easy
PARKING: Metered parking, though competitive (even on weekdays), is available throughout the area, including near the starting point of this walk on East First and Alameda Streets. Taking the train is recommended.
NEAREST METRO STATION: Metro's Gold Line serves this walk with the Little Tokyo/ Arts District station at the corner of East First and Alameda Streets, which is the starting point of the walk.

Like much of Los Angeles, the Arts District has undergone many changes over the last century and a half. And it continues to evolve to this day. Set alongside the LA River, the area had its modern roots in agriculture, first with wine grapes in the mid-19th century, then with citrus. A network of railroads was built to serve that industry, but as Los Angeles grew, the existing transportation infrastructure was ripe for the manufacturing era, giving rise to industrial buildings throughout the busy working-class district. But as trucking became an important part of goods shipment, the narrow streets and lack of space for larger factories kept the city from competing with newer industrial strongholds. Empty warehouses, though, were perfect for artists in need of large spaces starting in the 1970s, and the area later became an epicenter for street art. Today, however, the district is again in transition, with trendy shops, high-end art, and award-winning restaurants lining the streets.

Walk Description

Begin at the southeast corner at East First and Alameda Streets, across from the Little Tokyo/Arts District Metro station, and head south on Alameda. Situated between two freeways and home to Union Station a few blocks away (see Walk 29), this thoroughfare on the edge of downtown's core can be busy with traffic. This is also the future site of a small 1.9-mile underground rail infrastructure project that will have major implications for public transit. Once completed (slated for 2021 as of this writing), the Regional Connector Transit Project will allow for faster travel times across the county. Riders will be able to seamlessly travel between Pasadena and Long Beach or East LA and Santa Monica without ever having to leave their seats. Such a trip today involves three trains with two transfers.

After passing newer residential housing, hang a left on Traction Avenue. On the corner, at 216 S. Alameda St., sits ❶ **Angel City Brewery,** one of the larger brewery and public house spaces in the downtown area (it's also dog-friendly). This is the first taste you get of adaptive reuse on this walk. Some of the steel once produced in the 1913 building ended up on the Brooklyn Bridge and in Slinky toys. The architects, Hudson & Munsell, also designed the original Natural History Museum of LA County (see next walk), a few miles southwest.

Continue on Traction. When you hit the confluence with East Third Street, look up for a sign reading JOEL BLOOM SQUARE: ARTS DISTRICT PIONEER AND ACTIVIST. Bloom was the neighborhood's unofficial mayor who convinced the city to designate the area as the Arts District in the 1990s. Until his death, he operated Bloom's General Store around the corner.

Turn left onto East Third Street. Here, you find yourself among the latest transition into a trendy shopping district. At 800 E. Third St. is ❷ **Wurstküche,** a popular beer-and-brats spot that often has a line out the door. Farther down are clothing boutiques; ❸ **Salt & Straw**'s delectable ice cream from Portland, at 829 E. Third St.; and the fun art and lifestyle store ❹ **Poketo,** at 820 E. Third St. On the west side of the building housing Poketo, look up. Standing watch over the street is Shepard Fairey's *Peace Goddess,* painted in 2009. Fairey is best known as the artist behind the "Hope" poster from Barack Obama's 2008 presidential campaign.

Continue along East Third Street until you come upon the 900 block, where on the north side sits a large building with a handful of entrances to ❺ **Hauser Wirth & Schimmel,** a complex that holds art galleries, murals, an art-book store, a restaurant, a public garden, and a courtyard. Enter through the large entryway in the middle, and explore. This is the sixth complex by Hauser Wirth & Schimmel, the first of which opened in Switzerland in 1992. Exit the way you entered.

Turn left, continuing your journey two short blocks east on East Third Street until you hit Santa Fe Avenue. Stop and take in the imposing building across the street. Look left. Look right. You're in the middle of the quarter-mile-long, cruise ship–esque One Santa Fe, an apartment building with more than 400 units atop retail and businesses at the street level. "The design takes banality and stretches it like taffy in the direction of monumentality," noted the architecture critic at the *Los Angeles Times* when it opened in 2014.

Turn right to head south on Santa Fe Avenue. A courtyard within One Santa Fe will soon be visible on the left. Restaurants, grocery stores, and other shopping fill the space. Behind it, but out of view, is a Metro rail maintenance and storage yard that could be home to a new train station serving the Arts District. To your right is SCI-Arc, short for Southern California Institute of Architecture. Like its neighbor across the street, the college is a quarter mile long but was built more than 100 years ago as a freight house for the Atchison, Topeka, and Santa Fe Railroad.

Continue south along Santa Fe as it goes under the ramp to the Fourth Street Viaduct and bends right, becoming Mateo Street. Take Mateo as it again bends, this time to the left, and

Mural at the corner of Fifth and Colyton

continue south. This sleepier, more anonymous section gives a sense of what the Arts District used to be more like throughout.

After crossing Palmetto Street, an open-air shopping center named At Mateo aspires to become the focal point of the neighborhood. Under construction as of this writing, the complex, designed to fit the Arts District industrial aesthetic, is slated to open in late 2016. Across the street are numerous spots for eating and drinking: the vegetarian ❻ **Zinc Cafe** and its **Bar Mateo,** complete with one of the best alfresco spaces in the city; the popular San Francisco import ❼ **Blue Bottle Coffee;** and ❽ **The Spirit Guild,** a rare-vodka-and-gin tasting room.

At Sixth Street, turn right. Behind you is the site of the historic Sixth Street Viaduct, a former architectural gem that graced movies and TV throughout decades of pop culture. Unfortunately, the concrete employed when it was built in the 1930s deteriorated, leading to irreparable cracks. A replacement is expected to be completed in 2019.

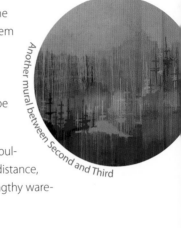
Another mural between Second and Third

Continue west on Sixth Street, where you'll pass LA Boulders, one of the city's popular climbing gyms. In the distance, the industrial roots of the neighborhood persist: a lengthy warehouse with long driveways for trucks to back into.

Turn left onto Mill Street and head to the aptly named Industrial Street.

Turn left on Industrial, where you'll enter another chic area of the district. At 1820 Industrial is ❾ **Daily Dose Cafe,** home to a cozy outdoor dining space in a narrow, curving alley with lights strung above. At 1850 Industrial is ❿ **Church & State,** often hailed as one of the best French restaurants in town. The eatery is located within the historic Biscuit Company Lofts (originally built for Nabisco) and across from the Toy Factory Lofts, both constructed in the mid-1920s.

Turn left here at Mateo, heading north back to Sixth Street, and retrace your steps to Palmetto, where you'll turn left.

Turn right at Hewitt Street. At 525 Hewitt St. is the LA Cleantech Incubator, a city-funded nonprofit to "accelerate development of cleantech start-ups." Companies that call it home run the gamut, from apps to lower your energy bills to solar tracking to indoor farming.

Continue down Hewitt to Fifth Street and turn left. On the corner, at 451 S. Hewitt St. is a location of the popular and expanding Urth Caffé chain.

Continue west on Fifth for one block, and turn right on Colyton.

On the corner, at 453 Colyton St., is the Arts District Co-op, a large, open warehouse space with an eclectic mix of businesses selling crafts and handpicked items. Continue north to Fourth Street.

Turn right on Fourth Street. Immediately on your right is the ⑪ **A+D Museum,** for architecture and design. This small museum has an especially focused mission: to exhibit progressive architecture and design in Los Angeles. To see the rotating exhibits, general admission is $7.

When Fourth Street hits Hewitt and Fourth Place, make a U-turn onto Fourth Place to head west. In a block, you'll again run into Hewitt. Turn right.

To your right is the entrance of ⑫ **Art Share L.A.** This nonprofit live/work space for up to 30 artists holds events and gallery viewing on its first floor. Stop in to check out the current gallery show and pick up a calendar of upcoming events. Continue northeast on Hewitt and turn left at Traction.

Now you're in for a treat. At 714 Traction Ave. is ⑬ **The Pie Hole,** one of the best spots in the city for pie. It's worth saving the appetite you've built up for this family-run spot that features a rotating selection of creative sweet and savory pies, such as Earl Grey tea, strawberry lavender, mac and cheese, and curry.

Continue along Traction, this time behind Wurstküche, until you arrive at Alameda. Turn right and walk one block to where you started.

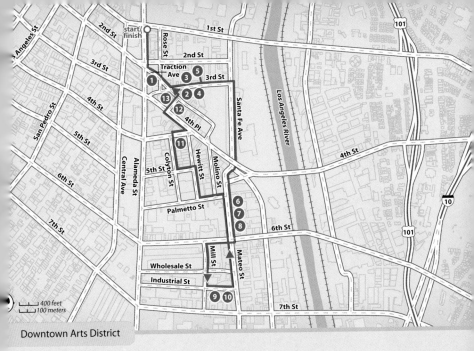

Downtown Arts District

Points of Interest

1. **Angel City Brewery** 216 S. Alameda St., Los Angeles, CA 90012; 213-622-1261, angelcitybrewery.com

2. **Wurstküche** 800 E. Third St., Los Angeles, CA 90013; 213-687-4444, wurstkuche.com

3. **Salt & Straw** 829 E. Third St., Los Angeles, CA 90013; 213-988-7070, saltandstraw.com

4. **Poketo** 802 E. Third St., Los Angeles, CA 90013; 213-537-0751, poketo.com

5. **Hauser Wirth & Schimmel** 901 E. Third St., Los Angeles, CA 90013; 213-943-1620, hauserworthschimmel.com

6. **Zinc Cafe/Bar Mateo** 580 Mateo St., Los Angeles, CA 90013; 323-825-5381, zinccafe.com

7. **Blue Bottle Coffee** 582 Mateo St., Los Angeles, CA 90013; bluebottlecoffee.com /cafes/arts-district

8. **The Spirit Guild** 586 Mateo St., Los Angeles, CA 90013; 213-613-2326, thespiritguild.com

9. **Daily Dose Cafe** 1820 Industrial St., Los Angeles, CA 90021; 844-932-4593, dailydosela.com

10. **Church & State** 1850 Industrial St., Los Angeles, CA 90021; 213-405-1434, churchandstatebistro.com

11. **A+D Museum** 900 E. Fourth St., Los Angeles, CA 90013; 213-346-9734, aplusd.org

12. **Art Share L.A.** 801 E. Fourth Place, Los Angeles, CA 90013; 213-687-4278, artsharela.org

13. **The Pie Hole** 714 Traction Ave., Los Angeles, CA 90013; 213-537-0115, thepieholela.com

Brilliantly colored specimens at the Exposition Park Rose Garden

34 USC and Exposition Park

BOUNDARIES: Figueroa St., Jefferson Blvd., Vermont Ave., Martin Luther King Jr. Blvd.
DISTANCE: About 1.5 miles
DIFFICULTY: Easy (includes short flights of steps)
PARKING: Metered parking is available on Exposition Blvd.
NEAREST METRO STATION: Exposition Park/USC

The University of Southern California is a world-renowned private learning institution with a state-of-the-art campus where students are extremely well cared for and at the same time held to very high expectations. The attractive college grounds are located south of downtown Los Angeles. Just across the street is Exposition Park, a state-owned property that is home to numerous museums and outdoor educational displays, the classically inspired Los Angeles Memorial Coliseum, and a magnificent rose garden (open all year, except during pruning in January and February).

Walk Description

Start on the west side of Figueroa Street at the intersection with Childs Way (just north of Exposition Boulevard). This is one of the entrances to the ❶ **USC campus.** Trojan Hall (a student residence) and the admissions office are located at 615 Childs Way. Walk west on Childs Way. At 635 is the Alumni House, a simple but elegant white clapboard building dedicated in 1880 as the original University of Southern California. According to the plaque in front of the structure, this is the oldest university building in all of Southern California.

Turn right to cut diagonally across the Alumni House plaza, heading northwest toward McCarthy Quad. You emerge into the expansive lawn area, where students gather to lounge around in the sun or frantically complete assignments on their laptops (the entire campus is equipped with wireless Internet access). The quad is bordered to the south by Doheny Library and to the north by Leavey Library—you can see the top of the Shrine Auditorium just beyond Leavey on the other side of Jefferson Boulevard.

Head west on Hellman Way, with Doheny Library on your left and the quad on your right. Pass Alumni Park on your left before coming to the very collegiate-looking (even by USC architectural standards) Bovard Administration Building. As you pass the north side of the building, you can even peek into the university president's opulent office, which occupies the northwest corner of the first floor. Next, you pass the renowned Annenberg School for Communication on your right and the Physical Education Building on your left.

Turn right just past the Annenberg building, and then turn left to enter Heritage Hall. In the lobby, you can admire every sports trophy USC has ever won, including countless Heisman Trophies awarded to the Trojan football team—quite impressive, if you're into that sort of thing.

Exit Heritage Hall and retrace your steps back along Hellman Way past Bovard; then turn right to cut diagonally across Alumni Park (heading southeast). Stop in the center of the park to admire the graceful Prentiss Memorial Fountain, also known as *Youth Triumphant* and *The Four Cornerstones of American Democracy.*

You'll have to circle the fountain to discover each of these cornerstone values; the words are engraved into the fountain and illustrated by pretty little statues.

Once through the park, turn left to head southeast on Childs Way. On your right, pass the Alfred Newman Recital Hall, which is decorated with an elaborate bas-relief of prehistoric mammals, and Hubbard Hall.

Turn right just past the entrance to Lewis Hall, following the brick-paved passage-way south toward Exposition Boulevard.

Exit through the gate onto Exposition Boulevard, and cross the street at the cross-walk before turning left toward Figueroa Street.

Turn right on Figueroa and continue to State Drive, where you'll turn right to enter Exposition Park. Suspended on your right is an old United Airlines jet—one of the Aerospace Museum's several outdoor air- and spacecraft displays.

As you continue west on State Drive, you pass the former Aerospace Museum (its future is unknown), which was designed by Frank Gehry in 1984.

Turn right just past the Aerospace Museum, passing the redbrick facade of the old Armory building, which is now home to the California Science Center's Annenberg wing.

The spectacular ❷ **Exposition Park Rose Garden** is on your left. Pause to admire the carefully ordered plots of colorful rosebushes, with the ornate domed building of the original Los Angeles County Historical and Art Museum (now part of the Natural History Museum) forming a picture-perfect backdrop. Walk through the garden toward the museum, breathing deeply to enjoy the sweetly scented air.

Emerge from the garden, and turn left. Then turn right at the next footpath, which you follow to the imposing entrance of the ❸ **Natural History Museum of Los Angeles County.** You can explore the grand interior architecture and educational displays of the museum for a moderate fee.

From the Natural History Museum entrance, follow the path south toward the Los Angeles Memorial Coliseum.

Turn left at the next path, and follow the walkway up into the remarkable plaza of the ④ **California Science Center.** This area is covered by a huge, cylindrical metal structure from which strings of gold balls hang, representing the galaxy. Admission to the Science Center's permanent exhibit galleries is free, so take some time to explore this truly educational and entertaining museum. The IMAX Theater is next door—if you have an extra hour or two and around $8 to spend, watching a film on one of the enormous screens is a sensory treat. After exploring the California Science Center, exit back out into the plaza and turn left (heading in the opposite direction of the Natural History Museum).

Just before you reach the parking structure adjacent to the IMAX Theater, turn right to follow the sidewalk, cross Exposition Park Drive, and then turn left on the other side of the street to head toward the main entrance of the ⑤ **Los Angeles Memorial Coliseum.** This 92,516-seat stadium held its first football game (USC versus Pomona College) in 1923 and has since hosted two Olympiads, two Super Bowls, and a World Series. Stop to check out the headless (and anatomically correct) statues of male and female Olympians in front of the stadium entrance.

Cross Exposition Park Drive once again to head back toward the parking structure, and then descend the staircase that leads into the sunken garden to the left of the structure.

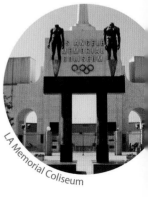

LA Memorial Coliseum

Follow the pleasant path past educational displays about hummingbirds and butterflies. An interactive exhibit on the top level of the parking structure shows kids how to use a lever to lift up an actual pickup truck—pretty cool. Continue to follow the path around the structure as it turns to the right, passing under an A-12 Blackbird spy craft built in the 1960s.

Ascend the stairs on your left and continue straight ahead, passing in front of the entrance to the ⑥ **California African American Museum.** If the museum is open, take advantage of the free admission to learn more about the cultural and artistic contributions that African Americans have made, particularly in California and the West.

When you find yourself back at the jet exhibit at the intersection of State Drive and Figueroa Street, exit Exposition Park onto Figueroa and turn left. Ahead, you'll see a giant neon sign for Felix Chevrolet/Cadillac, a pop culture landmark graced with the likeness of the lovable cartoon cat himself.

If you parked your car on Exposition Boulevard, turn left there or continue on Figueroa Street to the start of the walk at the intersection of Childs Way.

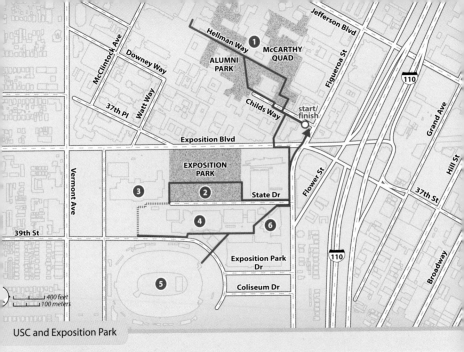

USC and Exposition Park

Points of Interest

1. **University of Southern California** Figueroa Street at Exposition Boulevard; usc.edu

2. **Exposition Park Rose Garden** 701 State Drive, Los Angeles, CA 90037; 213-763-0114, laparks.org/park/exposition-rose-garden

3. **Natural History Museum of Los Angeles County** 900 Exposition Blvd., Los Angeles, CA 90007; 213-763-3466, nhm.org

4. **California Science Center** 700 State Drive, Los Angeles, CA 90037; 323-724-3623 or 213-744-7400 (for IMAX Theater), californiasciencecenter.org

5. **Los Angeles Memorial Coliseum** 3911 S. Figueroa St., Los Angeles, CA 90037; 213-747-7111, lacoliseum.com

6. **California African American Museum** 600 State Drive, Los Angeles, CA 90037; 213-744-7432, caamuseum.org

Urban oasis: Elyria Canyon Park

35 Mount Washington

BOUNDARIES: Figueroa St., Cypress Ave., Division St., N. Ave. 50

DIRECTIONS: This route starts at the peak of Mount Washington, which can be tough to find. Follow these driving directions to successfully navigate the twists and turns of the narrow canyon roads:

*From the intersection of Figueroa St. and Marmion Way (**GPS: N34° 5.459' W118° 12.677'**), head north on Marmion Way. After 0.4 mile, turn left on W. Ave. 45. In 0.2 mile, bear right on Cañon Crest Ave. and, in another 0.2 mile, turn left on W. Ave. 46. Then, in 0.2 mile, turn left on Rome Dr. and follow it as it bends right; in another 0.2 mile, turn left on San Rafael Ave. Drive 1 block to arrive at the intersection of San Rafael and Elyria Dr.*

DISTANCE: 0.25 mile–1.5 miles, depending on route chosen

DIFFICULTY: Easy to strenuous (includes short flights of steps and optional dirt hiking trail)

PARKING: Free parking is available just inside the gates of the Self-Realization Fellowship.

Mount Washington is one of several idyllic communities hidden in the hills between downtown Los Angeles and Pasadena. This rustic neighborhood is populated with a collection of artistic, laid-back, nature-loving individuals, so it's no surprise that it's also home to the world headquarters of the Self-Realization Fellowship. Founded in 1920 by

Paramahansa Yogananda, this worldwide religious organization seeks to bring together people of all creeds in the pursuit of world peace and harmony—a noble goal, to be sure.

This walk can be whatever you want to make of it: either a short stroll through the grounds of the fellowship, where you can meditate on the beauty of your serene surroundings atop the hill and enjoy panoramic views of the city below, or a full-fledged hike that takes you from these carefully manicured grounds down through the rustic beauty of nearby Elyria Canyon Park and back up again.

Walk Description

Begin just inside the gates of the ❶ Self-Realization Fellowship International Headquarters, at the intersection of San Rafael Avenue and Elyria Drive. A small visitor center is just inside the gate to your left; here, you can speak to a volunteer or browse literature to learn more about this popular religious movement.

Head into the fellowship grounds, passing a large lawn area on your right before you come to a former tennis court. Descend the steps and cut lengthwise across the court. To your right is a sundial surrounded by benches—from here, you can sit and enjoy a view of the downtown high-rises a few miles south of Mount Washington.

Continue along the gravel path, which leads through a lush meditation garden of ferns, ficus trees, and palms. Private alcoves set back into the vegetation on either side of the path offer a place to contemplate or meditate; you'll be serenaded by the sound of a trickling fountain. Eventually, you come to a table and chairs carved out of stone that sit beneath a stand of pine trees—another lovely spot to stop for a rest, engage in deep thought, or stop thinking altogether.

Follow the path past the stone table and chairs as it turns left, ascend a short flight of steps, and take a quick right. Pass a planter filled with water and lily pads, and continue up the next set of steps, passing through a rose garden before you emerge back into the paved parking area.

Turn around here to head back toward the entrance to the fellowship. On your right is the main building: a distinctive three-story, flat-roofed structure established as the Mount Washington Inn, a popular resort for Hollywood stars and society types in the late 1800s and the early years of the 20th century. The Mount Washington Development Company even built a short railway leading up and down the hill to get patrons to and from the inn. The railway shut down long ago, but the former passenger depot still stands, down the hill at the corner of West Avenue 43 and Marmion Way.

Step inside the main building, which acts as the fellowship's headquarters, to check out the meditation chapel and Yogananda's library. After passing the former hotel, you reach a small gazebo on your right. Inside is a wishing well decorated with peaceful greetings and wishes from Yogananda himself.

If you wish, you can return to your car and end the walk. To keep going, exit the fellowship grounds and continue northwest on Elyria Drive, crossing San Rafael Avenue. A stunning shingled Craftsman home sits on the corner on your right.

Follow the road as it turns left. The chaparral-covered hills of Elyria Canyon slope down on your right. Continue all the way to the end of the street, where you arrive at a trailhead.

Follow the trail as it starts to descend through the grassy meadowland into the canyon. Thirty-five-acre ❷ **Elyria Canyon Park,** a Santa Monica Mountains Conservancy parkland, is home to one of the last remaining stands of California black walnut trees in greater Los Angeles. If you've brought your dog along for the hike, be sure to keep it leashed in the park. You should also watch out for poison oak, although you should be safe as long as you stick to the clearly marked trails.

When you come to the first split in the trail, take the right-hand path, which affords a view of Glendale in the distance.

At the next split, continue to follow your path as it curves to the right. The trail widens slightly here and shows remnants of asphalt paving. Continue downhill along the shady trail.

At the next split in the trail, follow the path that curves downhill to your left a short distance to the floor of the canyon and the Elyria Canyon Park entrance at Wollam Street.

Head back up the trail, bearing right at the split to continue along the same path you took down.

When you return to the point where the path widens, take the narrow dirt trail that branches off to the right instead of continuing back up the same trail you followed into the park. Follow this dirt trail as it curves left, affording a view of the other side of the canyon and the large homes perched high on the ridge above.

At the next split, take the narrow trail on the left that heads uphill and curves around through the bushes, past a bench and trash can, before it reconnects with your original path.

Turn right and take the trail back up to your starting point at the end of Elyria Drive.

Follow Elyria Drive back to the entrance of the Self-Realization Fellowship, where you began.

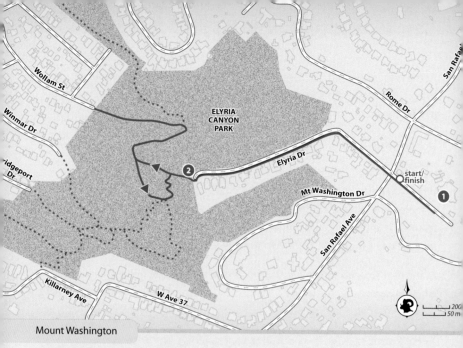

Points of Interest

1 Self-Realization Fellowship International Headquarters 3880 San Rafael Ave., Los Angeles, CA 90065; 323-225-2471, yogananda-srf.org

2 Elyria Canyon Park Dead end of Elyria Drive (main entrance: 1550 Bridgeport Drive), Los Angeles, CA 90065; tinyurl.com/elyriacanyon

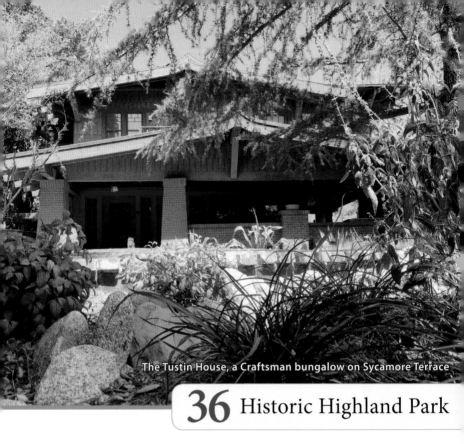

The Tustin House, a Craftsman bungalow on Sycamore Terrace

36 Historic Highland Park

BOUNDARIES: Marmion Way, N. Ave. 50, Griffin Ave., E. Ave. 43
DISTANCE: 2.5 miles
DIFFICULTY: Easy
PARKING: Near Marmion Way and Museum Dr.
NEAREST METRO STATION: Southwest Museum (Gold Line)

This large neighborhood of about 60,000 people on LA's northeast side has a long history. Located along a seasonal stream called the Arroyo Seco ("Dry River"), in a valley hugged by spring-fed rolling hills, Highland Park has always attracted residents, from its earliest native settlers, the Chumash, to later ones, who started America's Arts and Crafts movement here. The neighborhood is served by three rail stations, along with infrastructure that helped push the city's car-culture stereotype. CA 110, also known as the Arroyo Seco Parkway, was the first highway for automobiles in the country. Despite that, there are plenty of places that two feet will take you—as this walk will.

Walk Description

Begin at the Gold Line's Southwest Museum station, pragmatically named for the
① Historic Southwest Museum, around the corner at 234 Museum Drive. If you're
walking on a Saturday, stop by now or at the end of the walk if it's during visitor
hours (10 a.m.–4 p.m.; free admission). A satellite of The Autry Museum of the American West in Griffith Park, this museum was founded by Charles Lummis in 1907 as
the Southwest Museum of the American Indian (more on the eccentric Lummis
later). As the name indicates, it's dedicated to American Indian objects—so much so
that it's the second-largest collection in the country and widely revered.

Head south out of the Metro station to Woodside Drive and turn left onto the upper
(left) sidewalk at Figueroa Street. This sidewalk takes you above Figueroa and offers
your first glimpse of Highland Park's historic architecture. This is the Arts and Crafts
District, and you witness it immediately with the first house on the corner at
4601 N. Figueroa. This Queen Anne–American Craftsman hybrid is the Ziegler Estate,
bought by a former director of the Historic Southwest Museum to be added to the
museum's complex. Although its character is intact today, it is now a day care facility.

Next door, at 4605 N. Figueroa St., is Casa de Adobe, which is still owned by the
Historic Southwest Museum (but closed to the public). The house
looks like a Spanish California hacienda from the early 1800s,
but it was actually purpose-built in 1917 as a museum to
depict life under Spanish colonial rule. Before brick became
a dominant building material (though no longer, due to
earthquake regulations), adobe (mud brick) was a staple
building material across the American Southwest.

Continue down the sidewalk, noting several bungalows,
a quaint apartment building, and a couple of Craftsman
homes at 4665 and 4671 Figueroa.

Exhibits at the Historic Southwest Museum

Continue on the sidewalk until it spits you back onto Figueroa, and
go left. At the corner of Sycamore Terrace is the Hiner House, at 4757 Figueroa St.
Edward Hiner hailed from Kansas and founded the music department at the school

that eventually became UCLA. A friend of John Philip Sousa's (of "The Stars and Stripes Forever" fame), Hiner named his music studio, a building next to his mixed chalet/Tudor-style home, Sousa Nook. Sousa himself stayed there when he visited Hiner.

Take a left on Sycamore Terrace, being careful as you walk up this short, sidewalk-less section of the narrow street as it curves and inclines.

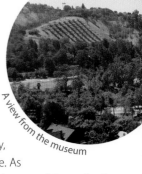

A view from the museum

As Sycamore straightens, you find yourself in the heart of the Arts and Crafts District: Professor's Row, named for the 15 years when Occidental College was nearby and its teachers resided here. The quaint Craftsman character remains throughout this block; several of the homes have been designated as Historic-Cultural Monuments by the city, including the Arroyo Stone House, at 4939 Sycamore Terrace. As the name indicates, the stones used to build this house (and many of the walls of the raised lawns at neighboring houses) were brought up from the Arroyo Seco.

When you come to North Avenue 50, turn right; then cross and turn right on Figueroa. You'll soon come upon two buildings owned by the Pillar of Fire Church, a Christian denomination with a half-dozen congregations around the country. (The organization's name comes from the Book of Exodus.)

Cross Avenue 49 into ❷ **Sycamore Grove Park.** Before it became a city park named after the native trees that shaded it, the grove in the late 1800s was known for rowdy picnicking fueled by alcohol. Today, it is a quiet, placid park with barbecue pits, a children's play area, picnic tables, tennis courts, and the Sousa-Hiner Bandshell, which sits in view of the aforementioned Hiner House across the street.

Behind the band shell, a path and a short tunnel lead to a pedestrian bridge across CA 110. When crossing above this busy artery, you'll notice that it looks different from most freeways. Its narrow lanes and the short, 90-degree on- and off-ramps can beget a nerve-wracking experience for drivers. The Arroyo Seco Parkway, as it is known, is the oldest freeway in the nation. It is also part of the official Route 66 alignment. As you finish crossing the freeway, you'll be above the 2-mile Arroyo Seco bike path.

The bridge will bring you to South Avenue 52. Turn right to follow the path leading away from the sidewalk and toward the bike path. Alternatively, this is the first of two opportunities for an optional detour. An entrance to the rolling hills of ❸ Ernest E. Debs Regional Park lies 0.1 mile straight ahead and on your left. A short distance up the driveway, you'll find the ❹ Audubon Center at Debs Park, where you can pick up a birding checklist and hiking-trail map.

Continue west on the shady Arroyo Seco Bike Path until you come to the parking lot of the Montecito Heights Recreation Center. This recreation facility is home to a senior center, a baseball diamond, and basketball courts, among other activity areas.

Walk through the parking lot to its south end, and turn right on Homer Street.

You're now in the small Montecito Heights neighborhood. The street is quaint, with a number of small Craftsman-inspired homes.

When you hit East Avenue 43, safely cross the street and arrive at your second choice of a side trip. For this optional detour, continue down Homer 0.3 mile to visit the ❺ Heritage Square Museum, a large, very cool outdoor museum where historic homes have been moved for preservation. Otherwise, take a right on East Avenue 43 to continue with this route.

After crossing CA 110 again, take a left on Carlota Boulevard to enter the grounds for the ❻ Charles Lummis Home and Gardens. Built of river rock and reminiscent of a fairy-tale cottage, this Craftsman beauty was the home of Charles Lummis, an eccentric Renaissance man who founded the Southwest Museum of the American Indian, walked across the country, fought for Indian rights, and so much more. You can explore this fascinating landmark,

Hiner House, 4757 Figueroa St.

usually open on weekends, on a free self-guided tour. When finished, head back the way you came to East Avenue 43, and take a left.

Arrive at Figueroa and go right two blocks, past numerous small businesses, until you reach West Avenue 45.

Take a left on West Avenue 45 and safely walk across the Metro Gold Line tracks, where you'll hit Marmion Way.

Go right on Marmion Way, and in less than 0.2 mile you'll be back at the Gold Line Station. If you haven't already, check out the Historic Southwest Museum around the corner.

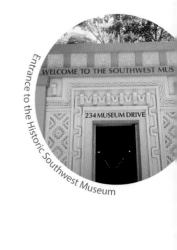

Entrance to the Historic Southwest Museum

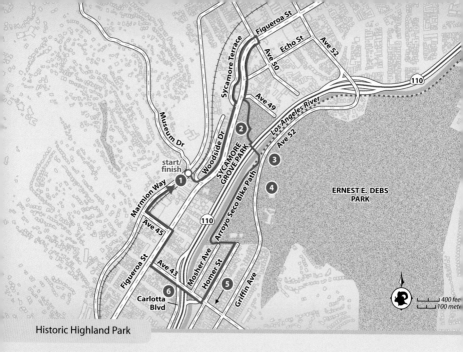

Points of Interest

1 **Historic Southwest Museum** 234 Museum Drive, Los Angeles, CA 90065; 323-495-4252, theautry.org/visit/mt-washington-campus

2 **Sycamore Grove Park** 4702 N. Figueroa St., Los Angeles, CA 90065

3 **Ernest E. Debs Regional Park** 4235 Monterey Road, Los Angeles, CA 90032

4 **Audubon Center at Debs Park** 4700 N. Griffin Ave., Los Angeles, CA 90031; 323-221-2255, debspark.audubon.org

5 **Heritage Square Museum** 3800 Homer St., Los Angeles, CA 90031; 323-225-2700, heritagesquare.org

6 **Charles Lummis Home and Gardens** 200 E. Ave. 43, Los Angeles, CA 90031; 323-661-9465, laparks.org/historic/lummis-home-and-gardens

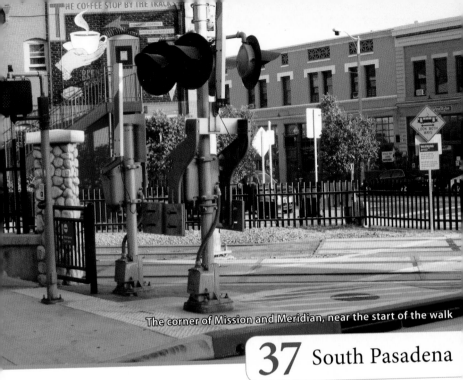

The corner of Mission and Meridian, near the start of the walk

37 South Pasadena

BOUNDARIES: Fair Oaks Ave., CA 110, Orange Grove Ave., El Centro St.
DISTANCE: About 1.25 mile
DIFFICULTY: Easy
PARKING: Free street parking is available on Meridian Ave., and there is a public parking
   structure on the corner of Meridian and Mission St.
NEAREST METRO STATION: Mission St. and Meridian Ave. (Gold Line)

A local store proprietor refers to South Pasadena as a "hipper Mayberry," and the description is apt. This city has a lovely, small-town sense of community, but at the same time it's fast becoming a happening shopping and dining destination.

This walk begins at the hub of "South Pas": Mission Meridian Village, an urban village centered around the Metro Gold Line station to reduce traffic and develop a community center by building housing within close proximity to public transportation and commercial attractions. Development around public-transit hubs has become a popular trend in Los Angeles within the decade, and the execution here is a successful example.

Walk Description

Begin at the corner of Hope Street and Meridian Avenue. The Mission Meridian complex's immaculate Craftsman duplexes line the west side of Meridian. Head south on Meridian, passing a boutique, a florist, and a public parking structure. ❶ **Heirloom Bakery & Cafe,** at 807 Meridian Ave., will no doubt tempt you with its scrumptious selection of goodies.

On the east side of Meridian, just before the railroad tracks, is a building sure to be of interest to movie buffs: a two-story Victorian cottage painted a pretty pale blue. Today it's an office building, but in 1978 it served as the home of the murderous Michael Myers in the original *Halloween*.

❷ **The Moo on Mission,** the second location of the popular Mother Moo Creamery out of Sierra Madre, sits in perfect view of the tracks, on the north-east corner of Mission and Meridian. Their small-batch, handcrafted sweets are definitely worth a try. Across the street, on the northwest corner, is a modern Indian restaurant housed in the former Mission Arroyo Hotel building, a South Pasadena cultural landmark.

When you reach Mission Street, turn right to find the crosswalk.

Cross to the south side of Mission Street at the crosswalk, and turn around to head east on Mission, toward the Metro station.

Turn right back onto Meridian. Pass a large woven-metal sculpture depicting, appropriately enough, a man walking. The ❸ **South Pasadena Historical Museum,** inside the Meridian Iron Works building at 913 Meridian, features exhibits depicting South Pasadena's history, beginning with the original American Indian residents, along with photos of the city during its early years of development. It's free to the public, so why not pop in and check it out? It's also worthwhile to cross to the island in the middle of the street to check out another cultural landmark, the ❹ **Watering Trough and Wayside Station,** which was erected in 1906 as a rest stop for horses and their riders. On the corner of Meridian Avenue and El Centro Street is ❺ **Bistro de la Gare,** a charming French-Italian restaurant and wine bar.

Turn right on El Centro to pass Nicole's Market & Café, a plant nursery, and the South Pasadena Gold Line station's south entrance.

Turn around to retrace your steps back to Meridian, and then continue east on El Centro. At 1009 El Centro is **6** **Communal Food & Drink,** a modern take on a beer garden. It's obvious that South Pasadena diners very much enjoy a tasty meal alfresco accompanied by a carefully matched drink. But then, who doesn't?

At 1019 El Centro, you pass the South Pasadena Bank Building, another cultural landmark; the two-story brick building now houses a hair salon and a coffee shop (South Pas dwellers appear to love their java, as well).

After crossing Diamond Avenue, you come to the South Pasadena Library Community Room, a distinguished brick-and-stone building set in a small, shady park. The city's Unified School District Administration building is on the opposite side of the street. (South Pasadena is known to lure young families away from the city of Los Angeles with its excellent school system.)

Continue on El Centro all the way to Fair Oaks Avenue, passing apartment buildings, the Fremont Centre Theatre, and a culinary arts school.

Turn left on Fair Oaks Avenue.

At the light, cross to the north side of Mission Street and turn left.

At 1526 Mission, **7** **Fair Oaks Pharmacy and Soda Fountain,** originally opened in 1915, offers a heavy dose of nostalgia with its tin ceilings, honeycomb-tile floors, and old-fashioned soda fountain. Stop in for a hand-dipped malt, egg cream, or lime rickey, and imagine what it was like when this served as a popular Route 66 pit stop.

At 1510 Mission, you reach **8** **Dinosaur Farm,** a toy store with a delightfully back-to-basics vibe that sells a terrific assortment of craft kits, musical instruments, games, and more. The store also offers story time and kids' classes in the back room.

As you continue west on Mission, you pass more clothing and home-interiors boutiques, antiques shops and other independent businesses; major chains are refreshingly few and far between in this part of town. Noteworthy stores include **9** **Marz,** a unique gift boutique at 1512, and **10** **Mission Wines,** at 1114.

At 1040 Mission, **11** **Mike & Anne's** offers delicious seasonal dishes with a gourmet flair on a welcoming patio. Across the street is Mission Street Yoga.

When you reach Meridian Avenue, turn right to return to your starting point at the corner of Hope Street.

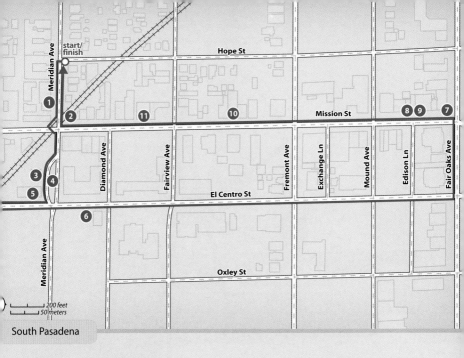

South Pasadena

Points of Interest

1 **Heirloom Bakery & Cafe** 807 Meridian Ave., South Pasadena, CA 91030; 626-441-0042

2 **The Moo on Mission** 1006 Mission St., South Pasadena, CA 91030; 626-441-0744, mothermoo.com

3 **South Pasadena Historical Museum** 913 Meridian Ave., South Pasadena, CA 91030; 626-799-9089

4 **Watering Trough and Wayside Station** Meridian Avenue just south of Mission Street, South Pasadena, CA 91030

5 **Bistro de la Gare** 921 Meridian Ave., South Pasadena, CA 91030; 626-799-8828, bistrodelagare.com

6 **Communal Food & Drink** 1009 El Centro St., South Pasadena, CA 91030; 626-345-5128, communalfoodanddrink.com

7 **Fair Oaks Pharmacy and Soda Fountain** 1526 Mission St., South Pasadena, CA 91030; 626-799-1414, fairoakspharmacy.net

8 **Dinosaur Farm** 1510 Mission St., South Pasadena, CA 91030; 626-441-2767, dinosaurfarm.com

9 **Marz** 1512 Mission St., South Pasadena, CA 91030; 626-799-4032, marzbazaar.com

10 **Mission Wines** 1114 Mission St., South Pasadena, CA 91030; 626-403-9463, missionwines.com

11 **Mike & Anne's** 1040 Mission St., South Pasadena, CA 91030; 626-799-7199, mikeandannes.com

An improvisational climbing structure near the Maritime Museum

38 San Pedro Waterfront

BOUNDARIES: Pacific Ave., Los Angeles Harbor, First St., Seventh St.
DISTANCE: About 1.5 miles
DIFFICULTY: Easy
PARKING: One-hour free parking is available in the lot for the battleship USS *Iowa* and Los Angeles Maritime Museum.

Due in large part to its coveted waterfront location and mild climate, LA's San Pedro district is ripe for gentrification. In recent years, the home of the Port of Los Angeles has been undergoing revitalization and redevelopment, including the relocation of the impressive Battleship USS *Iowa* naval warship—now open for tours—at Berth 87 and the addition of a picturesque waterfront promenade next door. Next up is a planned revamp of the kitschy and rundown Ports O' Call Village just south of the redesigned waterfront. Your best bet for visiting downtown San Pedro is during a First Thursday celebration, which features gallery openings, street vendors, and entertainment between 6 and 9 p.m. on the first Thursday of each month.

Walk Description

Begin south of First Street in the parking lot for the **❶ Battleship USS** *Iowa* and the **❷ Los Angeles Maritime Museum.** The Vincent Thomas Bridge and the loading cranes and shipping containers of the Port of Los Angeles create a colorful backdrop for the magnificent gray warship. Head away from the ship to reach the promenade walkway that runs alongside the parking lot, and then turn left to head south. The promenade has dancing fountains, benches, attractive landscaping, and even exercise equipment.

Soon you'll pass the fire boat station, which features a pleasant picnicking area and a giant ship's wheel out front.

As you step down to the wooden walkway alongside the docks, you'll notice a selection of enormous anchors on display to your right.

As you approach Sixth Street, you'll see the Downtown/Sixth Street stop for San Pedro's waterfront Red Car line. Until recently, this vintage electric trolley shuttled visitors between the World Cruise Center north of downtown and Ports O' Call Village to the south in replica railcars patterned after the 1909 Pacific Electric cars. At the time of this writing, the line had closed with plans to reopen as part of the Ports O' Call revitalization plan, but a free waterfront street trolley still runs during summer weekends (see sptrolley.com for details).

Take some time to explore the artifacts displayed in front of the Maritime Museum, including a ship's anchor and steering wheel, a memorial propeller from a World War II warship, and the front of the hull of the USS *Los Angeles.* If you have a few dollars and some extra time to spend, you can explore the museum itself, which boasts an impressive collection of ships, models, and navigational equipment, as well as rotating exhibits.

Turn right on Sixth Street. At the corner of Harbor and Sixth Street is the American Merchant Marine Veterans Memorial, which consists of a beautiful fountain sculpture by Jasper D'Ambrosi that depicts one man rescuing another from the sea. Follow Sixth Street west toward Old Historic San Pedro. The sidewalk on both sides of the street is lined with plaques for athletes and sports professionals who have some connection with either San Pedro or Los Angeles.

After crossing Centre Street, Sixth Street becomes trendier, featuring an assortment of boutiques, bistros, and breweries, as well as more-established businesses and art galleries housed in historic storefronts. The Art Deco ❸ **Warner Grand Theatre** is located at 478 W. Sixth St. The theater opened in 1931 and is on the National Register of Historic Places; today it serves as a venue for shows, concerts, and classic films.

Turn left on Pacific Avenue and walk one block.

Turn left on Seventh Street to enter the heart of the Downtown San Pedro Arts District, which features more galleries, shops, and eateries. This area also includes the inevitable upscale loft developments that show up in any burgeoning artists' community. The Bank Lofts in the historic Bank of San Pedro building are located at the corner of Mesa Street. Continue on Seventh Street all the way back to Harbor Boulevard.

Turn left on Harbor Boulevard to take a stroll through ❹ **John S. Gibson Memorial Park.** Owned by the Los Angeles Maritime Museum, the park is home to the American Merchant Marine Veterans Memorial as well as a striking Fishing Industry Memorial.

American Merchant Marine Veterans Memorial

Turn right when you reach Fifth Street to cut back into the waterfront promenade, and then turn left to follow the walkway back to your starting point in the USS *Iowa* parking lot.

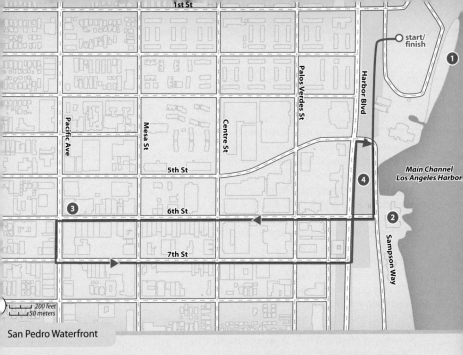

San Pedro Waterfront

Points of Interest

1 Battleship USS *Iowa* 250 S. Harbor Blvd., Los Angeles, CA 90731; 877-446-9261, pacificbattleship.com

2 Los Angeles Maritime Museum Berth 84 (foot of Sixth Street), San Pedro, CA 90731; 310-548-7618, lamaritimemuseum.org

3 Warner Grand Theatre 478 W. Sixth St., San Pedro, CA 90731; 310-548-2493, grandvision.org

4 John S. Gibson Memorial Park Harbor Boulevard between Fifth and Sixth Streets, San Pedro, CA 90731; 310-548-7618, lamaritimemuseum.org

Appendix 1: Walks by Theme

Architectural Tours

Arts and Culture

Dining, Shopping, and Entertainment

Appendix 2: Points of Interest

Beauty and Health

Aroma Spa and Sports 3680 Wilshire Blvd., Los Angeles, CA 90010; 213-387-0212, aromaresort.com (Walk 19, page 90)

Being in LA 2122 Hillhurst Ave., Los Angeles, CA 90027; 323-741-8035, beinginla.com (Walk 20, page 95)

dtox Day Spa 3206 Los Feliz Blvd., Los Angeles, CA 90039; 323-665-3869, dtoxdayspa.com (Walk 22, page 106)

Educational and Cultural Centers

Audubon Center at Debs Park 4700 N. Griffin Ave., Los Angeles, CA 90031; 323-221-2255, debspark.audubon.org (Walk 36, page 177)

Central Library 630 W. Fifth St., Los Angeles, CA 90071; 213-228-7000, lapl.org/central (Walk 31, page 150)

Go For Broke National Education Center 355 E. First St., Los Angeles, CA 90012; 310-328-0907, goforbroke.org (Walk 32, page 156)

The International School of Los Angeles 4155 Russell Ave., Los Angeles, CA 90027; 323-665-4526, internationalschool.la (Walk 21, page 102)

Japanese American Cultural and Community Center/James Irvine Japanese Garden 244 S. San Pedro St., Los Angeles, CA 90012; 213-628-2725, jaccc.org (Walk 32, page 156)

University of Southern California Figueroa Street at Exposition Boulevard; usc.edu (Walk 34, page 166)

Entertainment, Nightlife, and Performing Arts

El Portal Theatre 5269 Lankershim Blvd., North Hollywood, CA 91601; 213-480-3232, elportaltheatre.com (Walk 7, page 28)

Hollywood Bowl 2301 N. Highland Ave., Los Angeles, CA 90068; 323-850-2058, hollywoodbowl.com (Walk 15, page 69)

Kirk Douglas Theatre 9820 Washington Blvd., Culver City, CA 90232; 213-628-2772, centertheatregroup.org/visit/kirk-douglas-theatre (Walk 10, page 42)

Music Center (Dorothy Chandler Pavilion, Ahmanson Theatre, Mark Taper Forum, Walt Disney Concert Hall) 135 N. Grand Ave., Los Angeles, CA 90012; 213-972-7211, musiccenter.org (Walk 30, page 142)

NoHo Arts Center 11136 Magnolia Blvd., North Hollywood, CA 91601; 818-508-7101, thenohoartscenter.com (Walk 7, page 28)

Royce Hall, UCLA 340 Royce Drive, Los Angeles, CA 90095; 310-825-2101, roycehall.org (Walk 9, page 36)

The Satellite 1717 Silver Lake Blvd., Los Angeles, CA 90026; 323-661-4380, thesatellitela.com (Walk 25, page 118)

Two Roads Theater 4348 Tujunga Ave., Studio City, CA 91604; 818-415-9568, tworoadstheater.com (Walk 8, page 32)

Upright Citizens Brigade Theatre 5919 Franklin Ave., Los Angeles, CA 90028; 323-908-8702, ucbtheatre.com (Walk 16, page 75)

Warner Grand Theatre 478 W. Sixth St., San Pedro, CA 90731; 310-548-2493 (Walk 38, page 188)

Wiltern Theatre 3790 Wilshire Blvd., Los Angeles, CA 90010; 213-380-5005, wiltern.com (Walk 19, page 90)

Food and Drink

101 Coffee Shop 6145 Franklin Ave., Los Angeles, CA 90028; 323-467-1175, 101coffeeshop.com (Walk 16, page 75)

Akasha 9543 Culver Blvd., Culver City, CA 90232; 310-845-1700, akasharestaurant.com (Walk 10, page 42)

Alcove Cafe & Bakery 1929 Hillhurst Ave., Los Angeles, CA 90027; 323-644-0100 (Walk 20, page 95)

Angel City Brewery 216 S. Alameda St., Los Angeles, CA 90012; 213-622-1261, angelcitybrewery.com (Walk 33, page 160)

Aroma Coffee & Tea Company 4360 Tujunga Ave., Studio City, CA 91604; 818-508-0677, aromacoffeeandtea.com (Walk 8, page 32)

Back on the Beach Cafe 445 Pacific Coast Highway, Santa Monica, CA 90402; 310-393-8282, backonthebeachcafe.com (Walk 2, page 6)

BCD Tofu House 3575 Wilshire Blvd., Los Angeles, CA 90010; 213-382-6677, bcdtofu.com (Walk 19, page 90)

Beachwood Cafe 2695 N. Beachwood Drive, Los Angeles, CA 90068; 323-871-1717, beachwoodcafe.com (Walk 17, page 81)

Beachwood Market 2701 Belden Drive, Los Angeles, CA 90068; 323-464-7154 (Walk 17, page 81)

Birds 5925 Franklin Ave., Los Angeles, CA 90028; 323-465-0175, birdshollywood.com (Walk 16, page 75)

The Best Fish Taco in Ensenada 1650 N. Hillhurst Ave., Los Angeles, CA 90027; 323-466-5552, bestfishtacoinensenada.com (Walk 20, page 95)

Bistro de la Gare 921 Meridian Ave., South Pasadena, CA 91030; 626-799-8828, bistrodelagare.com (Walk 37, page 183)

Blue Bottle Coffee 582 Mateo St., Los Angeles, CA 90013; bluebottlecoffee.com /cafes/arts-district (Walk 33, page 160)

Bourgeois Pig 5931 Franklin Ave., Los Angeles, CA 90028; 323-464-6008 (Walk 16, page 75)

Brentwood Country Mart 225 26th St., Santa Monica, CA 90402; 310-451-9877 (Walk 3, page 10)

Caioti Pizza Cafe 4346 Tujunga Ave., Studio City, CA 91604; 818-761-3588, caiotipizzacafe.com (Walk 8, page 32)

Casa La Golondrina 17 Olvera St., Los Angeles, CA 90012; 213-628-4349 (Walk 29, page 135)

Church & State 1850 Industrial St., Los Angeles, CA 90021; 213-405-1434, churchandstatebistro.com (Walk 33, page 160)

Clifton's 648 S. Broadway, Los Angeles, CA 90014; 213-627-1673, cliftonsla.com (Walk 31, page 150)

Club Tee Gee 3210 Glendale Blvd., Los Angeles, CA 90039; 323-669-9631 (Walk 22, page 106)

Communal Food & Drink 1009 El Centro St., South Pasadena, CA 91030; 626-345-5128, communalfoodanddrink.com (Walk 37, page 183)

The Cook's Garden by HGEL 1033 Abbot Kinney Blvd., Los Angeles, CA 90291; 310-944-1151, groedibles.com (Walk 4, page 14)

Daily Dose Cafe 1820 Industrial St., Los Angeles, CA 90021; 844-932-4593, dailydosela.com (Walk 33, page 160)

The Dresden Restaurant 1760 N. Vermont Ave., Hollywood, CA 90027; 323-665-4294, thedresden.com (Walk 20, page 95)

Eat 11108 Magnolia Blvd., North Hollywood, CA 91601; 818-760-4787, eatnoho.com (Walk 7, page 28)

El Cóndor 3701 W. Sunset Blvd., Los Angeles, CA 90026; 323-660-4500, elcondorla.com (Walk 24, page 114)

Erewhon 7660 Beverly Blvd., Los Angeles, CA 90036; 323-937-0777, erewhonmarket.com (Walk 13, page 57)

Fair Oaks Pharmacy and Soda Fountain 1526 Mission St., South Pasadena, CA 91030; 626-799-1414, fairoakspharmacy.net (Walk 37, page 183)

Far East Plaza 727 N. Broadway, Los Angeles, CA 90012 (Walk 29, page 135)

Farmers Market 6333 W. Third St., Los Angeles, CA 90036; 323-933-9211, farmersmarketla.com (Walk 13, page 57)

The Federal Bar 5303 Lankershim Blvd., North Hollywood, CA 91601; 818-980-2555, thefederalbar.com (Walk 7, page 28)

Foo Chow Restaurant 949 N. Hill St., Los Angeles, CA 90012; 213-485-1294 (Walk 29, page 135)

Fred 62 1850 N. Vermont Ave., Los Angeles, CA 90027; 323-667-0062, fred62.com (Walk 20, page 95)

The Frog Spot 2825 Benedict St., Los Angeles, CA 90039; 323-223-0585, folar.org/frogspot (Walk 28, page 131)

Gjelina 1429 Abbot Kinney Blvd., Los Angeles, CA 90291; 310-450-1429, gjelina.com (Walk 4, page 14)

Grand Central Market 317 S. Broadway, Los Angeles, CA 90012; 213-624-2378 (Walk 30, page 142)

Heirloom Bakery & Cafe 807 Meridian Ave., South Pasadena, CA 91030; 626-441-0042 (Walk 37, page 183)

HMS Bounty 3357 Wilshire Blvd., Los Angeles, CA 90010; 213-385-7275 (Walk 19, page 90)

Honey's Kettle 9537 Culver Blvd., Culver City, CA 90232; 310-202-5453, honeyskettle.com (Walk 10, page 42)

Hop Louie 950 Mei Ling Way (inside Central Plaza), Los Angeles, CA 90012; 213-628-4244 (Walk 29, page 135)

India Sweets and Spices 3126 Los Feliz Blvd., Los Angeles, CA 90039; 323-345-0360, indiasweetsandspices.us (Walk 22, page 106)

Indochine Vien 3110 Glendale Blvd., Los Angeles, CA 90039; 323-667-9591, indochinevien.com (Walk 22, page 106)

Intelligentsia 3922 W. Sunset Blvd., Los Angeles, CA 90029; 323-663-6173, intelligentsiacoffee.com (Walk 24, page 114)

The Izaka-ya by Katsu-ya 1133 Highland Ave., Manhattan Beach, CA 90266; 310-796-1888, katsu-yagroup.com/manhattan-beach (Walk 6, page 24)

The Kettle 1138 Highland Ave., Manhattan Beach, CA 90266; 310-545-8511, thekettle.net (Walk 6, page 24)

LA Mill 1636 Silver Lake Blvd., Los Angeles, CA 90026; 323-663-4441, lamillcoffee.com (Walk 25, page 118)

La Poubelle 5907 Franklin Ave., Los Angeles, CA 90028; 323-465-0807, lapoubellebistro.com (Walk 16, page 75)

Larchmont Farmers Market 209 N. Larchmont Blvd., Los Angeles, CA 90004; Sundays, 10 a.m.–2 p.m. (Walk 18, page 86)

Lemonade 1661 Abbot Kinney Blvd., Los Angeles, CA 90291; 310-452-6200, lemonadela.com/locations/westside/venice (Walk 4, page 14)

Le Pain Quotidien 8607 Melrose Ave., West Hollywood, CA 90069; 310-854-3700, lepainquotidien.com/store/melrose (Walk 12, page 52)

Le Petit Greek 127 N. Larchmont Blvd., Los Angeles, CA 90004; 323-464-5160, lepetitgreek.com (Walk 18, page 86)

Mike & Anne's 1040 Mission St., South Pasadena, CA 91030; 626-799-7199, mikeandannes.com (Walk 37, page 183)

Millie's 3524 W. Sunset Blvd., Los Angeles, CA 90026; 323-664-0404, milliescafela.com (Walk 24, page 114)

Molly Malone's Irish Pub 575 S. Fairfax Ave., Los Angeles, CA 90036; 323-935-1577, mollymalonesla.com (Walk 13, page 57)

The Moo on Mission 1006 Mission St., South Pasadena, CA 91030; 626-441-0744, mothermoo.com (Walk 37, page 183)

Palermo Ristorante Italiano 1858 N. Vermont Ave., Los Angeles, CA 90027; 323-663-1178, palermorestaurant.net (Walk 20, page 95)

Pazzo Gelato 3827 W. Sunset Blvd., Los Angeles, CA 90026; 323-662-1710 (Walk 24, page 114)

Philippe the Original 1001 N. Alameda St., Los Angeles, CA 90012; 213-628-3781, philippes.com (Walk 29, page 135)

The Pie Hole 714 Traction Ave., Los Angeles, CA 90013; 213-537-0115, thepieholela.com (Walk 33, page 160)

Pine & Crane 1521 Griffith Park Blvd., Los Angeles, CA 90026; 323-668-1128, pineandcrane.com (Walk 24, page 114)

Pitfire Pizza Company 5108 Lankershim Blvd., North Hollywood, CA 91601; 818-980-2949 (Walk 7, page 28); 108 W. Second St., Los Angeles, CA 90012; 213-808-1200 (Walk 30, page 142); pitfirepizza.com

Prado Restaurant 244 N. Larchmont Blvd., Los Angeles, CA 90004; 323-467-3871, pradola.com (Walk 18, page 86)

Republic of Pie 11118 Magnolia Blvd., North Hollywood, CA 91601; 818-308-7990, republicofpie.com (Walk 7, page 28)

Salt & Straw 240 N. Larchmont Blvd., Los Angeles, CA 90004, 323-466-0485 (Walk 18, page 86); 829 E. Third St., Los Angeles, CA 90013, 213-988-7070 (Walk 33, page 160); saltandstraw.com

Shake Shack 8520 Santa Monica Blvd., West Hollywood, CA 90069; 323-488-3010, shakeshack.com/location/west-hollywood (Walk 12, page 52)

The Spirit Guild 586 Mateo St., Los Angeles, CA 90013; 213-613-2326, thespiritguild.com (Walk 33, page 160)

Spitfire Grill 3300 Airport Ave., Santa Monica, CA 90405; 310-397-3455, spitfiregrill.net (Walk 5, page 23)

Spoke Bicycle Cafe 3050 N. Coolidge St., Los Angeles, CA 90039; 323-684-1130, spokebicyclecafe.com (Walk 28, page 131)

Surfas Culinary District 8777 Washington Blvd., Culver City, CA 90232; 310-559-4770, surfasonline.com (Walk 10, page 42)

Sweetie Pie's NoHo 5230 Lankershim Blvd., North Hollywood, CA 91601; 818-761-1325, sweetiepiesnoho.com (Walk 7, page 28)

Sweet Lady Jane 1631 Montana Ave., Santa Monica, CA 90403; 310-254-9499, sweetladyjane.com (Walk 3, page 10)

Tacos Villa Corona 3185 Glendale Blvd., Los Angeles, CA 90039; 323-661-3458 (Walk 22, page 106)

Tam O'Shanter Inn 2980 Los Feliz Blvd., Los Angeles, CA 90039; 323-664-0228, lawrysonline.com/tam-oshanter (Walk 22, page 106)

The Tasting Kitchen 1633 Abbot Kinney Blvd., Los Angeles, CA 90291; 310-392-6644, thetastingkitchen.com (Walk 4, page 14)

Tender Greens 9523 Culver Blvd., Culver City, CA 90232; 310-842-8300, tinyurl.com /tendergreenscc (Walk 10, page 42)

Tokyo Delve's Sushi Bar 5239 Lankershim Blvd., North Hollywood, CA 91601; 818-766-3868, tokyodelvessushirestaurant.com (Walk 7, page 28)

Trois Familia 3510 W. Sunset Blvd., Los Angeles, CA 90026; 323-725-7800, troisfamilia.com (Walk 24, page 114)

Uncle Bill's Pancake House 1305 Highland Ave., Manhattan Beach, CA 90266; 310-545-5177, unclebills.net (Walk 6, page 24)

Urth Caffé 8565 Melrose Ave., West Hollywood, CA 90069; 310-659-0628, urthcaffe.com (Walk 12, page 52)

Venice Farmers Market Corner of Dell Avenue and South Venice Boulevard, Los Angeles, CA 90291; Fridays, 7–11 a.m. (Walk 4, page 14)

Village French Bakery 1414 W. Kenneth Road, Glendale, CA 91201; 818-241-2521 (Walk 23, page 110)

Village Pizzeria 131 N. Larchmont Blvd., Los Angeles, CA 90004; 323-465-5566, villagepizzeria.net (Walk 18, page 86)

Vitello's Italian Restaurant 4349 Tujunga Ave., Studio City, CA 91604; 818-769-0905, vitellosrestaurant.com (Walk 8, page 32)

Wurstküche 800 E. Third St., Los Angeles, CA 90013; 213-687-4444, wurstkuche.com (Walk 33, page 160)

Zinc Cafe/Bar Mateo 580 Mateo St., Los Angeles, CA 90013; 323-825-5381, zinccafe.com (Walk 33, page 160)

Historical Landmarks and Monuments

Avila Adobe 10 Olvera St., Los Angeles, CA 90012; 213-628-1274 (Walk 29, page 135)

Barnsdall Art Park/Hollyhock House 4800 Hollywood Blvd., Los Angeles, CA 90027; 323-644-6269 (Walk 20, page 95)

Bradbury Building 304 S. Broadway, Los Angeles, CA 90012 (Walk 30, page 142)

Charles Lummis Home and Gardens 200 E. Ave. 43, Los Angeles, CA 90031; 323-661-9465, laparks.org/historic/lummis-home-and-gardens (Walk 36, page 177)

City Hall 200 N. Spring St., Los Angeles, CA 90012; 213-473-7001, lacity.org (Walk 30, page 142)

The Ebell of Los Angeles 743 S. Lucerne Blvd., Los Angeles, CA 90005; 323-931-1277, ebellla.org (Walk 18, page 86)

Ennis House 2607 Glendower Ave., Los Angeles, CA 90027 (Walk 20, page 95)

Go For Broke Monument 160 N. Central Ave., Los Angeles, CA 90012 (Walk 32, page 156)

Los Angeles Theatre 615 S. Broadway, Los Angeles, CA 90014; 213-629-2939, losangelestheatre.com (Walk 31, page 150)

Union Station 800 N. Alameda St., Los Angeles, CA 90012; metro.net/about/union-station (Walk 29, page 135)

Watering Trough and Wayside Station Meridian Avenue just south of Mission Street, South Pasadena, CA 91030 (Walk 37, page 183)

Hotels

The Culver Hotel 9400 Culver Blvd., Culver City, CA 90232; 310-558-9400, culverhotel.com (Walk 10, page 42)

The Line Hotel 3515 Wilshire Blvd., Los Angeles, CA 90010; 213-381-7411, thelinehotel.com (Walk 19, page 90)

Millennium Biltmore Hotel 506 S. Grand Ave., Los Angeles, CA 90071; 213-624-1011, tinyurl.com/millenniumbiltmorela (Walk 31, page 150)

Westin Bonaventure Hotel 404 S. Figueroa St., Los Angeles, CA 90071; 213-624-1000, westin.com/bonaventure (Walk 31, page 150)

Museums and Galleries

A+D Museum 900 E. Fourth St., Los Angeles, CA 90013; 213-346-9734, aplusd.org (Walk 33, page 160)

América Tropical Interpretive Center 125 Paseo De La Plaza, Los Angeles, CA 90012; 213-628-1274, theamericatropical.org (Walk 29, page 135)

Art Share L.A. 801 E. Fourth Place, Los Angeles, CA 90013; 213-687-4278, artsharela.org (Walk 33, page 160)

Battleship USS *Iowa* 250 S. Harbor Blvd., Los Angeles, CA 90731; 877-446-9261, pacificbattleship.com (Walk 38, page 188)

The Broad 221 S. Grand Ave., Los Angeles, CA 90012; 213-232-6200, thebroad.org (Walk 30, page 142)

California African American Museum 600 State Drive, Los Angeles, CA 90037; 213-744-7432 (Walk 34, page 166)

California Science Center 700 State Drive, Los Angeles, CA 90037; 323-724-3623 or 213-744-7400 (for IMAX Theater), californiasciencecenter.org (Walk 34, page 166)

Fowler Museum at UCLA 308 Charles E. Young Drive N., Los Angeles, CA 90024; 310-825-4361, fowler.ucla.edu (Walk 9, page 36)

The Geffen Contemporary at MOCA 152 N. Central Ave., Los Angeles, CA 90013; 213-625-4390, moca.org/visit/geffen-contemporary (Walk 32, page 156)

Hauser Wirth & Schimmel 901 E. Third St., Los Angeles, CA 90013; 213-943-1620, hauserworthschimmel.com (Walk 33, page 160)

Heritage Square Museum 3800 Homer St., Los Angeles, CA 90031; 323-225-2700, heritagesquare.org (Walk 36, page 177)

Historic Southwest Museum 234 Museum Drive, Los Angeles, CA 90065; 323-495-4252, theautry.org/visit/mt-washington-campus (Walk 36, page 177)

Hollywood Heritage Museum 2100 N. Highland Ave., Hollywood, CA 90068; 323-874-4005, hollywoodheritage.org (Walk 15, page 69)

Japanese American National Museum/National Center for the Preservation of Democracy 100 N. Central Ave., Los Angeles, CA 90012; 213-625-0414, janm.org (Walk 32, page 156)

Los Angeles County Museum of Art 5905 Wilshire Blvd., Los Angeles, CA 90036; 323-857-6000, lacma.org (Walk 13, page 57)

Los Angeles Maritime Museum Berth 84 (foot of Sixth St.), San Pedro, CA 90731; 310-548-7618, lamaritimemuseum.org (Walk 38, page 188)

Museum of Contemporary Art 250 S. Grand Ave., Los Angeles, CA 90012; 213-626-6222, moca.org (Walk 30, page 142)

Museum of Flying 3100 Airport Ave., Santa Monica, CA 90405; 310-398-2500, museumofflying.org (Walk 5, page 23)

Natural History Museum 900 Exposition Blvd., Los Angeles, CA 90007; 213-763-3466, nhm.org (Walk 34, page 166)

Old Plaza Firehouse 501 N. Los Angeles St., Los Angeles, CA 90012; 213-485-8437 (Walk 29, page 135)

Pacific Design Center and MOCA 8687 Melrose Ave., West Hollywood, CA 90068; 310-657-0800, pacificdesigncenter.com (Walk 12, page 52)

La Brea Tar Pits Museum/Hancock Park 5801 Wilshire Blvd., Los Angeles, CA 90036; 323-934-7243, tarpits.org (Walk 13, page 57)

Schindler House/MAK Center for Design 835 N. Kings Road, West Hollywood, CA 90069; 323-651-1510, makcenter.org (Walk 12, page 52)

South Pasadena Historical Museum 913 Meridian St., South Pasadena, CA 91030; 626-799-9089 (Walk 37, page 183)

Parks and Gardens

Airport Park 3201 Airport Ave., Santa Monica, CA 90405 (Walk 5, page 23)

Annenberg Community Beach House 415 Pacific Coast Highway, Santa Monica, CA 90402; 310-458-4904, annenbergbeachhouse.com (Walk 2, page 6)

Baldwin Hills Scenic Overlook 6300 Hetzler Road, Culver City, CA 90232 (Walk 11, page 48)

Brand Park 1601 W. Mountain St., Glendale, CA 91201; 818-548-3782, tinyurl.com/brandpark (Walk 23, page 110)

Carthay Circle Park Commodore Sloat Drive north to Wilshire Boulevard, Los Angeles, CA 90048 (Walk 14, page 64)

Culver City Park 9910 Jefferson Blvd., Culver City, CA 90232 (Walk 10, page 42)

Echo Park and Echo Park Lake 751 Echo Park Ave., Los Angeles, CA 90026; 213-847-0929 (Walk 26, page 123)

Elysian Park 929 Academy Road, Los Angeles, CA 90012; 213-485-5054, laparks.org/park /elysian (Walk 27, page 128)

Elyria Canyon Park dead end of Elyria Drive (main entrance: 1550 Bridgeport Drive), Los Angeles, CA 90065; tinyurl.com/elyriacanyon (Walk 35, page 172)

Ernest E. Debs Regional Park 4235 Monterey Road, Los Angeles, CA 90032 (Walk 36, page 177)

Exposition Park Rose Garden 701 State Drive, Los Angeles, CA 90037; 213-763-0114, laparks.org/park/exposition-rose-garden (Walk 34, page 166)

Franklin D. Murphy Sculpture Garden Charles E. Young Drive E., Los Angeles, CA 90095; 310-443-7000, tinyurl.com/murphysculpturegarden (Walk 9, page 36)

Grand Park 200 N. Grand Ave., Los Angeles, CA 90012; grandparkla.org (Walk 30, page 142)

Hancock Park/La Brea Tar Pits and Museum 5801 Wilshire Blvd., Los Angeles, CA 90036; 323-934-7243, tarpits.org (Walk 13, page 57)

John S. Gibson Memorial Park Harbor Boulevard between Fifth and Sixth Streets, San Pedro, CA 90731; 310-548-7618, lamaritimemuseum.org (Walk 38, page 188)

Kings Road Park 1000 N. Kings Road, West Hollywood, CA 90069 (Walk 12, page 52)

Mar Vista Recreation Center 11430 Woodbine St., Los Angeles, CA 90066; 310-398-5982, laparks.org/reccenter/mar-vista (Walk 5, page 23)

Marsh Park 2944 Gleneden St., Los Angeles, CA 90039; 310-589-3200, tinyurl.com /marshparkla (Walk 28, page 131)

Mildred E. Mathias Botanical Garden 777 Tiverton Drive, UCLA, Los Angeles, CA 90095; 310-825-1260, botgard.ucla.edu; call ahead (Walk 9, page 36)

Palisades Park Ocean Avenue between Colorado Avenue and Adelaide Drive, Santa Monica, CA 90402 (Walk 2, page 6)

Pan Pacific Park and Recreation Center 7600 Beverly Blvd., Los Angeles, CA 90036; 323-939-8874, laparks.org/reccenter/pan-pacific (Walk 13, page 57)

Sand Dune Park Bell Avenue, Manhattan Beach, CA 90266; 310-802-5410 (Walk 6, page 24)

Silver Lake Recreation Center 1850 Silver Lake Blvd., Los Angeles, CA 90026; 323-644-3946 (Walk 25, page 118)

Sycamore Grove Park 4702 N. Figueroa St., Los Angeles, CA 90065 (Walk 36, page 177)

Syd Kronenthal Park 3459 McManus Ave., Culver City, CA 90232 (Walk 11, page 48)

Westminster Off-Leash Dog Park 1234 Pacific Ave., Los Angeles, CA 90291; 310-310-1550, venicedogpark.org (Walk 4, page 14)

Woodbridge Park 11240 Moorpark St., Studio City, CA 91602; 11240 Moorpark St., Studio City, CA 91602; 818-769-4415, laparks.org/park/woodbridge (Walk 8, page 32)

Shopping

Ackerman Union/UCLA Store 308 Westwood Plaza, Los Angeles, CA 90095; 310-825-7711, asucla.edu/student-union (Walk 9, page 36)

Brentwood Country Mart 225 26th St., Santa Monica, CA 90402; 310-451-9877, brentwoodcountrymart.com (Walk 3, page 10)

Counterpoint Records & Books 5911 Franklin Ave., Los Angeles, CA 90028; 323-957-7965, counterpointla.com (Walk 16, page 75)

Dinosaur Farm 1510 Mission St., South Pasadena, CA 91030; 626-441-2767, dinosaurfarm.com (Walk 37, page 183)

The Grove 189 The Grove Drive, Los Angeles, CA 90036; 888-315-8883, thegrovela.com (Walk 13, page 57)

Japanese Village Plaza 335 E. Second St., Los Angeles, CA 90012; japanesevillageplaza.net (Walk 32, page 156)

Marz 1512 Mission St., South Pasadena, CA 91030; 626-799-4032, marzbazaar.com (Walk 37, page 183)

Mel & Rose 8344 Melrose Ave., West Hollywood, CA 90069; 323-655-5557, melandrose.com (Walk 12, page 52)

Mission Wines 1114 Mission St., South Pasadena, CA 91030; 626-403-9463, missionwines.com (Walk 37, page 183)

Saigon Plaza 800 N. Broadway, Los Angeles, CA 90012 (Walk 29, page 135)

Samy's Camera 431 S. Fairfax Ave., Los Angeles, CA 90036; 323-938-2420, samys.com (Walk 13, page 57)

Potted 3158 Los Feliz Blvd., Los Angeles, CA 90039; 323-665-3801, pottedstore.com (Walk 22, page 106)

Poketo 802 E. Third St., Los Angeles, CA 90013; 213-537-0751, poketo.com (Walk 33, page 160)

Skylight Books 1818 N. Vermont Ave., Los Angeles, CA 90027; 323-660-1175, skylightbooks.com (Walk 20, page 95)

Surfas Culinary District 8777 Washington Blvd., Culver City, CA 90232; 310-559-4770, surfasonline.com (Walk 10, page 42)

Surplus Value Center 3828 W. Sunset Blvd., Los Angeles, CA 90026; 323-662-8132, surplusvaluecenter.net (Walk 24, page 114)

Yolk 1626 Silver Lake Blvd., Los Angeles, CA 90026; 323-660-4315, shopyolk.com (Walk 25, page 118)

Spiritual Institutions

Cathedral of Our Lady of Angels 555 W. Temple St., Los Angeles, CA 90012; 213-680-5200, olacathedral.org (Walk 30, page 142)

Lake Shrine Temple, Self-Realization Fellowship 17190 Sunset Blvd., Los Angeles, CA 90272; 310-454-4114, yogananda-srf.org (Walk 1, page 2)

Self-Realization Fellowship International Headquarters 3880 San Rafael Ave., Los Angeles, CA 90065; 323-225-2471, yogananda-srf.org (Walk 35, page 172)

Vedanta Society of Southern California 1946 Vedanta Place, Hollywood, CA 90068; 323-465-7114, vedanta.org (Walk 16, page 75)

Wilshire Boulevard Temple 3663 Wilshire Blvd., Los Angeles, CA 90010; 213-388-2401, wbtla.org (Walk 19, page 90)

Miscellaneous

Academy of Television Arts and Sciences 5220 Lankershim Blvd., North Hollywood, CA 91601; 818-754-2800, emmys.com/academy (Walk 7, page 28)

Brady Bunch House 11222 Dilling St., Studio City, CA 91604 (Walk 8, page 32)

Bunche Hall, UCLA 11282 Portola Plaza, Los Angeles, CA 90095 (Walk 9, page 36)

Castillo del Mar (former Thelma Todd House) 17531 Posetano Road, Los Angeles, CA 90272 (Walk 1, page 2)

Conjunctive Points Hayden Avenue between Higuera Street and National Boulevard, Culver City, CA 90232 (Walk 11, page 48)

The Culver Studios 9336 Washington Blvd., Culver City, CA 90232; 310-202-1234, theculverstudios.com (Walk 10, page 42)

Former John Barrymore House 17501 Castellammare Drive, Los Angeles, CA 90272 (Walk 1, page 2)

Los Angeles Memorial Coliseum 3911 S. Figueroa St., Los Angeles, CA 90037; 213-747-7111, lacoliseum.com (Walk 34, page 166)

Los Feliz Municipal Golf Course 3207 Los Feliz Blvd., Los Angeles, CA 90039; 323-663-7758, golf.lacity.org/cdp_los_feliz.htm (Walk 22, page 106)

Manhattan Beach Pier/Roundhouse Aquarium Western end of Manhattan Beach Blvd., Manhattan Beach, CA 90266; 310-379-8117 (Walk 6, page 24)

Margaret Herrick Library, Academy of Motion Picture Arts and Sciences 333 S. La Cienega Blvd., Beverly Hills, CA 90211; 310-247-3020, oscars.org/library (Walk 14, page 64)

Shakespeare Bridge Franklin Avenue at Monon Street, Los Angeles, CA 90027 (Walk 21, page 102)

West Hollywood Library 625 N. San Vicente Blvd., West Hollywood, CA 90069; 310-652-5340, colapublib.org/libs/whollywood (Walk 12, page 52)

Index

Page references followed by *p* indicate a photo;
those followed by *m* indicate a map.